Himalayan Salt

and

Himalayan Salt Lamps

William Cook

Himalayan Salt and Himalayan Salt Lamps

To my amazing wife
and our two wonderful daughters.
All that I do is done for you.

Table of Contents

Introduction

Salt is essential for life. We simply cannot <u>exist</u> without it.

However, there is a massive difference between conventional refined table salt and natural, unrefined, health-promoting salt… and it's essential to know and understand that difference.

In which case…

Welcome to the world of Himalayan salt and Himalayan salt lamps.

Within this book you will discover all there is to know about this unique, natural substance.

The health benefits that can be derived from the use of Himalayan salt are manyfold, and this book will take you on a journey to a greater understanding of this life-enhancing product and, ultimately, better health.

Salt is something that most people take for granted, it's just "there", it's accepted as is and regarded by most as somewhat unremarkable. However, the truth is that salt is an essential part of life and is a major player in our overall health.

Too little and we're in trouble, too much and we're possibly in even bigger trouble.

It's remarkable to think that such a simple, seemingly insignificant substance like salt has such an impact on your overall health, but it does.

Fortunately, people are becoming more and more aware of the dangers that are associated with consuming too much salt. There are numerous newspaper articles, radio discussions, TV items etc., warning of the potential dangers of high salt intake and the medical community is concerned about the impact that it can have upon a person's health, and they are right to be concerned.

However, too little salt will also lead to health complications because of its role in almost every function of the human body.

When the water and salt balance in the body are compromised, be it too much or too little of either, you're in trouble.

However, there are different types of salt, and it's safe to say that as far as the end product that finally resides on our dining table is concerned, not all salts are created equally.
Some salts are more beneficial than others and at the head of the table (pun entirely intended!) is Himalayan salt.

Why? Because it is a completely natural substance that hasn't been stripped of any of its inherent natural properties that are of almost immeasurable benefit to us.

It is salt as nature intended it to be.

We have been told for years that higher than recommended intake of regular table salt can contribute towards a number of health issues, including damage to our heart and raising blood pressure. Consequently, many of us are actively looking for ways to limit our salt intake as part of our pursuit of a healthier lifestyle.

However, Himalayan salt is different from other salts.

Regular table salt has been processed to the point that it is hardly recognizable as being a derivative of the original substance from which it started. Himalayan salts, on the other hand, undergo NO processing and, therefore, retain all of their original minerals and nutrients, and have <u>nothing</u> added to them.

Some people say that the difference between ordinary table salt and Himalayan salt is as great as the difference between white sugar lumps and a freshly cut sugar cane. The heavily processed end product bearing little resemblance to the original.

This analogy between table salt and white sugar has even more poignancy when you consider the fact that processed sugar is nowadays considered by most health professionals as a real and present danger to our wellbeing.

If you are low on any of the minerals that your body needs in order to function properly, then various health issues can quickly ensue, but with Himalayan salt, you may be able to rebalance their respective optimum levels.

For those who are worried about consuming too much salt via their diet, there are other ways that you will be able to reap the benefits of Himalayan salts without relying on diet alone, including salt baths and salt inhalers.

We'll look at Himalayan salt origins, properties, structure, and obviously, its health benefits, and we'll discuss the differences between Himalayan salt and ordinary table salt.

Need a unique gift? There are some really great gift ideas... and we'll be looking at cooking on a salt block!

Himalayan salt lamps are probably the easiest way to benefit from some of the myriad positives that come from using this unique product. They are easy to incorporate into any room, be it in your home or office, with a choice of colours and sizes to greatly enhance the aesthetics of the room in which they are placed.

Himalayan Salt and Himalayan Salt Lamps

We'll discuss the health benefits of Himalayan salt lamps, how to make sure that you purchase a genuine lamp in a buyer's guide, and much more!

It's going to be a fun and informative journey, so let's get started!

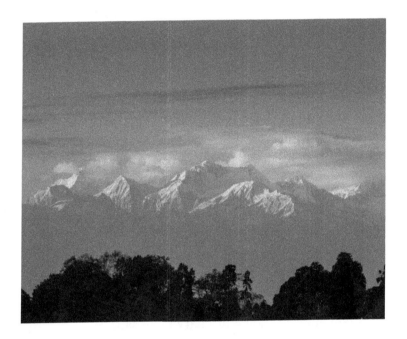

Some Interesting Salt Facts

For millennia, indeed as far back as 6050 BC, salt has been an integral and important part of the world's history and the development of civilizations. Great importance has been placed upon salt as a commodity, even the word "salary" being derived from the word "salt". It was of such importance that its production was actually restricted in ancient times to keep its value high, as it was used as currency and a method of trade.

Salt's ability to preserve food was a major contributory factor in the development of many civilizations, as it helped to eliminate dependence on the seasonal availability of food and made it possible for food to be shipped long distances over long periods of time.

As far back as 2700 BC, a writing on pharmacology was published in China and a great degree of that document is devoted to a discussion about more than 40 kinds of salt. Indeed, the Chinese government realised that taxing salt would be a particularly viable source of revenue for them.

Moving from China to Greece, the term "not worth his salt" comes from the practice of exchanging slaves for quantities of salt and by the time of the late Roman Empire and throughout the middle ages, salt was a highly valued, indeed precious commodity that was carried along salt roads.

Salt was carried and used by early explorers as a bargaining tool and has been used extensively in religious ceremonies throughout the world; indeed there are more than 30 references to salt in the Bible, one of which being the well-known phrase "the salt of the earth".

Himalayan Salt and Himalayan Salt Lamps

For a period of time in the 16th century, the world mistakenly started to consider rock salt as inferior to sea salt and as a result, a vast kingdom within Poland that had been built around the sale of rock salt collapsed.

In the mid 1700s, the British aristocrat, Lord Howe, was elated by his success of capturing General Washington's salt supply and India's Mahatma Gandhi defied the then British laws on salt to gain popular support.

During the American Civil War, President Davis offered immunity of military service to anybody who would look after salt production, as not only was it used in a dietary capacity, but it was also vital for tanning leather, preserving meat and in dyeing cloth for uniforms.

When the Dutch managed to blockade the Iberian salt works, it lead directly to Spanish bankruptcy.

In North America, the very first patent issued by the British government to an American settler was indeed for the exclusive rights for his particular method of salt production.

Moorish merchants of the 6th century regularly traded, weight for weight, equal amounts of salt for gold. So back in those days, salt was "worth its weight in gold"... literally!

In the UK, whole areas of Cheshire are renowned for salt production and actually led to the small port of Liverpool becoming a huge city, built largely upon the exporting of salt during the 19th century.

Venice rose to be an economic powerhouse due to salt production, and no prizes for guessing where the name Salzburg in Austria came from - it literally means "city of salt".

Some Interesting Salt Facts

Talking of Venice, in 1295, having returned home from his travels, Venetian explorer, Marco Polo, told how he had come across highly valued coins made of salt and still bearing the seal of Genghis Khan, the long deceased leader of the Mongolian Empire.

In total, a quarter of a billion tons of all types of salt is mined each year throughout the world, with 40% being produced by the United States and China.

In many cultures, salt is thought to be a source of power to drive away evil spirits and it is the custom in some European countries to throw a handful of salt into the coffin before burial because salt is seen as a symbol of immortality.

Salt is so vital to our existence that cells in the tongue are dedicated to its detection.

In Britain, any place name with the suffix "wich" means that it was once a source of salt, as in, for example, Nantwich or Norwich.

Crystal salt, as Himalayan salt is, used to be called "King Salt" because it was reserved for the exclusive use of royalty and the nobility.

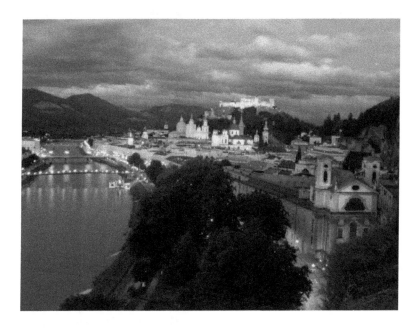

The beautiful city of Salzburg, Austria

Chapter 1: Himalayan Salt

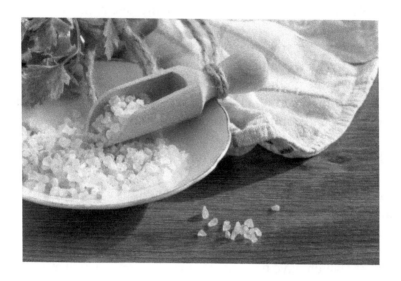

In the pursuit of a healthier lifestyle, there's an almost bewildering amount of information - and misinformation - about every aspect of health and well-being to be found on every platform known to man! Be it magazines, radio, TV, online, newspaper articles by the dozen, or just general workplace chat, we are almost on a daily basis bombarded with facts and figures about what's good or not good for you.

However, if you are looking for something that is easy to incorporate into your daily routine, has many significant health benefits and is a completely natural product void of any processing, then you will want to take a look at Himalayan salts.

I think it would be wise at this point to explain a little about the science behind the benefits that are derived from the use of Himalayan salt, as I'm of the opinion that it is better for everyone when thinking about embarking on a new health regime or trying to improve well-being in any way to fully understand the principles and processes by which this improvement can be made.

The very fact that you have purchased this book shows you have an inquisitive and enquiring mind and that you wish to further your knowledge on this particular subject and, as such, the understanding of certain principles will go a great way towards a more secure and comfortable process of improvement.

So, here we go with the science bit!...

Everything in the universe, from a mountain, to you and I, to the water in the oceans and the air that we breathe, is made up of molecules and atoms. Atoms are themselves made out of three types of particles; protons (which are positively charged), neutrons (which have no charge), and electrons (which are negatively charged). A molecule is electrically neutral - a point that shall become relevant later.

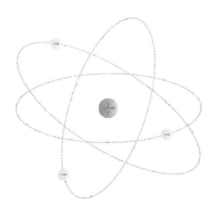

Chapter 1: Himalayan Salt

Protons and neutrons form the positively charged central core of an atom called the nucleus and, if you wish, imagine electrons as orbiting the nucleus like moons around a planet. At times, and during certain chemical processes, an electron will leave its orbit around the nucleus. When this happens, it turns the previously electrically neutral molecule into what is called a "positively charged ion".

Due to nature's inherent wish for balance, this ion will try any way it can to replace the missing electron, even if that means "stealing" it from another molecule. Because of differences in molecular structure, which include differences in how strong the bond is between an electron and its nucleus and the number of electrons in the outer orbits, some substances lose electrons more easily than others. Therefore, the positively charged ion will have greater or lesser difficulty in replacing its missing electron by taking (stealing) it from one of those different substances.

Obviously, this is a simplification of what is a fairly complex concept, but its relevance will easily become apparent as you get further into the book as we start discussing the various ways of using Himalayan salt, and the resulting relevant health benefits, some of which will be as a direct result of the interplay between positive and negative ions.

Himalayan salt is an unprocessed, pure form of salt that retains all the original elements, minerals, and nutrients that salt is supposed to have.

How it all came about

The Himalayan Mountains stand at a site that was once a primordial sea, and within that ancient, primal body of water, there existed a perfect ecosystem.

The sea eventually evaporated under the intense heat of the sun and as it receded, it left behind its rich, life-giving minerals in the form of deep veins of salt.

Over millions of years, the earth's tectonic plates moved, and at the junction of the Indian and Eurasian plates, a grindingly slow, but nonetheless immensely powerful collision took place, which resulted in the mountain range of the Himalayas being born, as each tectonic plate pushed unforgivingly against the other, forcing the land mass to climb higher and higher into the air.

Himalayan salt, formed over 250,000,000 years ago and free from all pollutants, is now mined from deposits in the foothills of the Salt Range hill system at the Khewra Salt Mine in Jhelum, part of the Punjab region of Pakistan. It's the world's oldest and second largest salt mine and attracts up to 275,000 visitors per year.

Known locally over hundreds of years for its preventative and restorative effect on the human body, it has been hand-mined and used by the people of the Himalaya region for centuries and is still a major part of their indigenous culture.

It is pure, unadulterated salt presented to you and I in its perfect form:- nothing added, nothing taken away.

Let's take a look at Himalayan salt and how it differs from regular table salt and why it's actually good for your health.

Himalayan salt vs. table salt

Himalayan salt is identical in composition to the ancient primal oceans and contains all the trace elements and minerals that occur naturally in the human body.

Chapter 1: Himalayan Salt

Table salt is basically a mixture of sodium and chloride, with all the beneficial compounds stripped from the original substance during its processing. Very often, salt companies will mine poor quality rock salt in order to keep costs down and this is then heated in kilns to about 1200 degrees Fahrenheit, which actually changes its chemical structure and destroys all the trace minerals and elements. A whole host of additives, including anti-caking agents, fluoride, and synthetic iodine are then thrown into the mix. These additives also include ferrocyanide and silica alumina. Ferrocyanides have been shown to damage our kidneys and aluminate consumption has been associated with numerous neurological disorders.

It must be said that problems associated with salt consumption is a relatively new phenomena, but this is down to the fact that not only are we using refined table salt to put ONTO our food, but also, it is being put INTO our food, in particular being added in excessive amounts to processed foods. **You don't even need to add salt to your food to be taking in too much in the first place, as it's been estimated that 75% of the salt we eat is by way of consuming everyday foods such as ready meals, breakfast cereals, and bread.**

The minerals that were an intrinsic part of the structure of the salt, and that keep blood pressure in balance, have been stripped from the original substance, which leads to refined table salt causing significant elevations in blood pressure, and we all know that having high blood pressure (hypertension) can lead to many life-threatening health conditions and complications, including heart attacks, aneurysms, kidney disease, peripheral artery disease, and eye damage.

There are many scientists and nutritionists who are now of the opinion that the body actually sees table salt as a toxin, and therefore, it places a massive strain on the body systems as they try to deal with this alien substance.

It's a well known and long established fact that too much sodium in the diet can lead to significant health issues and when you consider how much sodium can be consumed inadvertently by way of its presence as an additive in a multitude of products, including some we wouldn't even <u>think</u> would contain salt, it's no wonder that these health issues are becoming more and more prevalent in today's society.

If you're wondering <u>why</u> newly mined salt would be stripped of its beneficial minerals in the first place, and it's certainly something I asked myself many years ago, the answer lies in the fact that only 7% of the salt produced is intended for human consumption, the other 93% goes to industry which requires a more chemically pure sodium chloride, as this is what's used in the manufacture of chlorine gas, explosives, plastics, and fertilizers.

So, in effect, ordinary table salt is nothing more than an industrial bi-product, where its safety for human consumption is merely an afterthought, because apparently you and I come further down the list of priorities when compared to profit.

Himalayan salt has 84 natural trace elements and minerals and its pink colour is due to the presence of iron oxide, concentration levels of which can vary resulting in different shades of salt, from almost white to a deep orange.

You may be thinking that you've been hearing for years that salt is bad for you and indeed, it can be a contributory factor in weight gain, increased blood pressure, raising the risk of stroke, heart disease, kidney issues, water retention and the resulting bloating, and more. While having a little bit of salt is fine, most people in advanced "Western" cultures will get 2-3 times the amount of sodium that they need in their diets <u>each day.</u>

Chapter 1: Himalayan Salt

So why are many health professionals now recommending Himalayan salt to help <u>improve</u> your health?

In particular, salt provides us with two elements, sodium and chloride. Both of these elements are _essential_ for life and the body cannot make these elements by itself, so they must be obtained via the diet.

Himalayan salt, as well as other unprocessed sea salts, contains approximately 84% sodium chloride, of which just under 37% is pure sodium. Processed table salt, however, contains approximately 97.5% sodium chloride, of which just over 39% is pure sodium.

Although at first there appears to be little difference in those numbers as regards sodium, remember that the human body reacts intensely to even the slightest change in level or ratio of any essential element on which it depends.

For thousands of years, salt in general was known as a panacea, with many physicians from antiquity referring to it as "the fifth element". Himalayan salt that comes hand-mined naturally from the earth contains a great many beneficial nutrients that help the body function properly.

Himalayan salt is presented in its original, natural form, free from processing and just like nature intended salt to be. Indeed, it remains just as it was millions of years ago, without any pollutants.

On the other hand, table salt has been processed to the point whereby nearly all of those naturally occurring, beneficial nutrients are gone, mainly due to the intense heat treatment that table salt is subjected to during its processing.

So you end up with a product that is <u>very</u> different from its original form, because not only has table salt been stripped of the original beneficial minerals, but also chemicals are <u>added</u> to it.

At this point, it must be said that…

<u>The blood pressure stabilising effect of Himalayan salt, by way of its trace minerals, can only be achieved if the level of table salt AND salt as a hidden additive in other foods is reduced.</u>

In other words, if you reduce your table salt intake and the intake of salt as a food additive, then Himalayan salt can do its work properly and greatly aid in the many functions of the body, including the actual lowering and stabilising of blood pressure.

It is the author's belief that the food industry, with its introduction of low-sodium foods, has created a whole new market for itself in an attempt to address a problem that itself was created by the very same food corporations.

By stripping all the naturally occurring minerals from organic salt, then adding toxic chemicals to form table salt, and also "hiding" salt in so many foods that the average person wouldn't even realise contained salt in the first place, they tragically created a health epidemic and, surprise-surprise, came up with a, for them, very profitable solution to a problem of their own making.

Processed foods are nearly always very high in sodium content and it is always in the form of refined table salt/canned salt, with artificial flavours and flavour enhancers thrown in for good measure. It is bizarre and indeed very disturbing that many low-sodium products often contain the compound monosodium glutamate, which is itself a sodium-based product that has been shown to be a possible cause of heart attacks in individuals who don't have enough magnesium in their system. The magnesium they need is readily available in organic vegetables and Himalayan salt.

If you want to cut down on your sodium levels and overall salt intake, then drastically cut back on snacks and pre-prepared meals, as these are, by a long, long way, the greatest source of hidden salts in our diet. Always read the label, as you might be surprised at the level of salt in some products and even more surprised that other products contain any kind of salt in the first place!

It is a popularly held belief that table salt is just sodium chloride, but it isn't. Compounds are added to it to make it more free-flowing. Those compounds can include ferrocyanide, talc, and silica aluminates. Aluminium, present in the body through salt intake and through the use of aluminium-based deodorants and antiperspirants and absorbed through the skin, can lead to neurological disorders.

This is particularly so if there is not enough selenium in the body to help chelate the aluminium (attach to it) prior to expulsion. Another problem associated with insufficient levels of selenium is that the aluminium bioaccumulates (absorbed into the tissues faster than it can be expelled) over a period of time, which causes further degeneration.

Talc is a well known carcinogen, yet it is regularly added to table salt. Why the food industry has so scant regard for the well-being of its customers/consumers as is clearly shown with practices such as this and others, is a mystery. It appears as though they just don't care, as long as it makes their products nice to look at and easy to package.

Although there hasn't been a great deal of investigation into the effects of ingested talc, it has been banned from being used in other products, such as baby powders, because of the known health risks. However, and this is crazy but true, the use of talc in table salt is permitted, even though it is prohibited in all other foods because of its known toxicity and carcinogenic properties.

A scary fact is that table salt can contain up to 2% talc.

As a point of interest, unrefined Himalayan salt and sea salt contain more iodine than iodized table salt. In fact, a more accurate term would be sodium iodide, because iodide is iodine that has been combined with salt (sodium). Not only that, but with an irony that if it wasn't so tragic it'd be laughable, the added iodide found in table salt is of nowhere near the same benefit to the body as the iodide naturally found in Himalayan salt, because table salt has had all the very trace minerals removed that are necessary for the proper absorption of the iodide to occur in the first place!

It is worth mentioning that sodium alone without other minerals and trace elements present, as is the case with normal table salt, will not provide adequate cellular hydration either, because, once again, the very minerals and trace elements that are missing are those that are vital for this process to occur properly.

Indeed, sodium consumed in isolation may actually deplete other minerals from the body and so it is vitally important that we take in salt in its holistic form. Calcium, magnesium, and potassium are needed in the exact proportions as they appear in natural salt, so that our body can fully absorb and optimally utilize all the inherent trace elements and minerals.

Chapter 2: Himalayan Salt Spectral Analysis

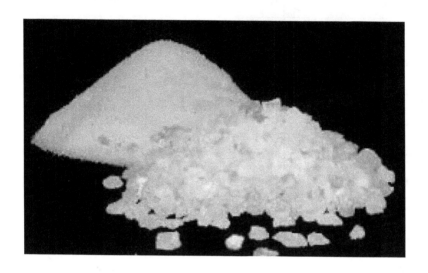

The table below shows the results for spectral analysis of a typical sample of Himalayan salt. It lists ALL minerals, elements, and electrolytes that are to be found in Himalayan salt.

Element	Ion	Concentration
Actinium	Ac	<0.001 ppm
Aluminium	Al	0.661 ppm
Antimony	Sb	<0.01 ppm
Arsenic	As	<0.01 ppm
Astatine	At	<0.001 ppm
Barium	Ba	1.96 ppm

Himalayan Salt and Himalayan Salt Lamps

Beryllium	Be	<0.01 ppm
Bismuth	Bi	<0.10 ppm
Boron	B	<0.001 ppm
Bromine	Br	2.1 ppm
Cadmium	Cd	<0.01 ppm
Calcium	Ca	4.05 g/kg
Carbon	C	<0.001 ppm
Cerium	Ce	<0.001 ppm
Cesium	Cs	<0.001 ppm
Chloride	Cl	590.93 g/kg
Chromium	Cr	0.05 ppm
Cobalt	Co	0.60 ppm
Copper	Cu	0.56 ppm
Dysprosium	Dy	<4.0 ppm
Erbium	Er	<0.001 ppm
Europium	Eu	<3.0 ppm
Fluoride	F	<0.1 g
Francium	Fr	<1.0 ppm
Gadolinium	Gd	<0.001 ppm
Gallium	Ga	<0.001 ppm
Germanium	Ge	<0.001 ppm
Gold	Au	<1.0 ppm

Hafnium	Hf	<0.001 ppm
Holmium	Ho	<0.001 ppm
Hydrogen	H	0.30 g/kg
Indium	In	<0.001 ppm
Iodine	I	<0.1 g
Iridium	Ir	<2.0 ppm
Iron	Fe	38.9 ppm
Lanthanum	La	<0.001 ppm
Lead	Pb	0.10 ppm
Lithium	Li	0.40 g/kg
Lutetium	Lu	<0.001 ppm
Magnesium	Mg	0.16 g/kg
Manganese	Mn	0.27 ppm
Mercury	Hg	<0.03 ppm
Molybdenum	Mo	0.01 ppm
Neodymium	Nd	<0.001 ppm
Neptunium	Np	<0.001 ppm
Nickel	Ni	0.13 ppm
Niobium	Nb	<0.001 ppm
Nitrogen	N	0.024 ppm
Osmium	Os	<0.001 ppm
Oxygen	O	1.20 g/kg

Palladium	Pd	<0.001 ppm
Phosphorus	P	<0.10 ppm
Platinum	Pt	0.47 ppm
Plutonium	Pu	<0.001 ppm
Polonium	Po	<0.001 ppm
Potassium	K	3.5 g/kg
Praseodymium	Pr	<0.001 ppm
Promethium	Pm	Unstable artificial isotope
Protactinium	Pa	<0.001 ppm
Radium	Ra	<0.001 ppm
Rhenium	Re	<2.5 ppm
Rhodium	Rh	<0.001 ppm
Rubidium	Rb	0.04 ppm
Ruthenium	Ru	<0.001 ppm
Samarium	Sm	<0.001 ppm
Scandium	Sc	<0.0001 ppm
Selenium	Se	0.05 ppm
Silicon	Si	<0.1 g
Silver	Ag	0.031 ppm
Sodium	Na	382.61 g/kg
Strontium	Sr	0.014 g/kg
Sulphur	S	12.4 g/kg

Tantalum	Ta	1.1 ppm
Technetium	Tc	Unstable artificial isotope
Tellurium	Te	<0.001 ppm
Terbium	Tb	<0.001 ppm
Thallium	Ti	0.06 ppm
Thorium	Th	<0.001 ppm
Thulium	Tm	<0.001 ppm
Tin	Sn	<0.01 ppm
Titanium	Ti	<0.001 ppm
Uranium	U	<0.001 ppm
Vanadium	V	0.06 ppm
Wolfram	W	<0.001 ppm
Ytterbium	Yb	<0.001 ppm
Yttrium	Y	<0.001 ppm
Zinc	Zn	2.38 ppm
Zirconium	Zr	<0.001 ppm

NB The above list contains not only the "84 trace minerals" as is often referred to in scholarly articles, but also elements and electrolytes.

Obviously, some of these minerals appear in Himalayan salt as miniscule amounts, but as previously mentioned, the human body reacts significantly to even the tiniest variations in the levels of certain elements, with scientists measuring the optimal amounts of certain substances in micrograms. So with many of the elements that our body needs, it's a case of a tiny amount can make a big difference

Upon reading the list of elements and minerals found in the spectral analysis of Himalayan pink salt, the reader may be somewhat alarmed to see certain words springing out from the text; words such as "lead" and "plutonium", so let me address this.

As can be seen in the list, analysis of pink Himalayan salt has shown it to contain a concentration level of 0.10 parts per million (the equivalent of 100 parts per billion) of lead, which is actually only one fifth of the legal limit for food. It has to be pointed out that lead is present in many other foodstuffs as a natural constituent and in quantities many, many times greater than the 100 parts per billion (ppb) shown to be in Himalayan salt.

Lead is a naturally occurring metal within the earth's crust and it is found naturally in water, soil, and even in the air that we breathe. Soil that is classed as _uncontaminated_ contains lead concentrations of not greater than 50,000 ppb. Compare that with many urban areas whose soil exceeds 200,000 ppb.

The World Health Organisation's maximum acceptable level of lead in water is 10 ppb, which equates to approximately 20 μg (micrograms) of lead if you were to drink 2 litres of water.

Conversely, if you consume 6g of pink Himalayan salt, which is the maximum daily amount of salt that should be consumed for optimal effect, you will have only taken in 0.6 μg of lead. So you can see how the lead content of Himalayan salt is negligible and is of no consequence to health and well-being, particularly when compared to the relatively vast quantities of lead consumed by the intake of other foodstuffs.

Chapter 2: Himalayan Salt Spectral Analysis

And here's the really interesting part; in an analysis of 13 top quality gourmet salts, they found that the majority of those salts contained approximately 500 ppb of lead. One particular sea salt from France contained 1300 ppb of lead. And, critically, regular table salt has on average 440 ppb of lead. One particular study showed that lead in regular table salt from some mines in Iran ranged anywhere from 430 ppb to 1520 ppb, and those figures are actually consistent with lead levels in table salt from several other countries. These averages, therefore, are way higher than the 100 ppb of lead found during the analysis of Himalayan salt.

On average, an adult can take in anywhere from 15µg to 240 µg of lead per day. The European Food Safety Authority (EFSA) conducted a detailed study of lead levels within various foods and their conclusion was that the level of lead, even in ordinary table salt, was of no significance. They found that all wheat grains contained up to 47 ppb of lead, all vegetables contained up to 92 ppb, all seafood contained up to 104 ppb, table salt was up to 278 ppb, meat contained 273 ppb, spices contained up to 364 ppb, and wild pigs (?!) contained 687,000 ppb of lead.

In all, 14.1% of over 700 foods sampled contained more than 10,000 ppb of lead!

The EFSA also found that potatoes, beer, and even tap water contained levels of lead hundreds of times more than normal table salt. Milk, coffee, and bottled water also contained many, many more times the level of lead found in Himalayan salt.

Wine, chocolate, rice, and tea also contained vastly greater quantities of lead than Himalayan salt.

So it's easy to see why the food authorities consider the naturally occurring lead found in normal salt to be of no significance and add to that the fact that levels of lead in Himalayan salt are even lower.

So, to put it into perspective, if you were to stop having salt, be it conventional table salt or Himalayan salt, due to concerns over lead consumption, you would also have to stop eating vegetables, as they all contain far higher levels of lead.

It is worth pointing out here that, of course, the symbol < means "less than" and therefore a reading of < 0.001 ppm means exactly that - there is less than 0.001 ppm contained within the sample, so there could in reality be only 0.0001ppm or even 0.00001ppm.

And now onto the plutonium content...

It is actually a very similar story to that of lead, because trace quantities of plutonium are present naturally in the environment, and the human body has always had a base load of natural plutonium.

Natural plutonium is created when uranium, which is present in abundance throughout the earth's crust, undergoes a process called "spontaneous fission" which leads directly to the formation of trace quantities of natural plutonium.

Himalayan salt comes from the mining of deposits whose veins were formed more than 250 million years ago, and obviously, has never been exposed to man-made radiation. There is natural radiation in every mine everywhere on Earth, in fact, there is natural radiation all around us, including its presence in water, soil, and all foods. The measurement of less than 1 ppb of natural plutonium in Himalayan salt is of no consequence whatsoever.

Conventional table salt, as has been discussed, undergoes many processes such as extreme heat treatment, bleaching, chemical cleaning, and the adding of iodine and anti-caking substances, which can include toxic ingredients like aluminium and ferrocyanide. Also, a small amount of sugar or corn syrup is added to disguise the taste of the anti-caking additive and to help preserve any added iodine.

All in all, these substances add up to being around 2% of the overall constituents of table salt. This 2% represents a level of approximately 20,000,000 ppb!

That's 20 million parts per billion of stuff that was <u>never</u> meant to be in salt in the first place, as opposed to 1 part per billion of something that has been there for the past 250 million years and occurs naturally in the earth's crust anyway.

I once read a great little article that talked about how apricots contain a very small amount of natural fluoride, which, of course, poses no health risk, but the vast quantities of fluoride added to water <u>is</u> a health risk because Mother Nature NEVER intended us to drink water with high levels of fluoride in it!

Himalayan salt is a complete, unrefined, synergistically balanced package, just as nature always intended it to be.

One final, but very important point before we move on to the next section is that the elements found within Himalayan salt are integrated into the salt's crystal grid. This is a vital, inherent property because it means that those elements are biomechanically available to our cells, due to the fact that they occur in an ional-colloidal form.

This is important to mention as it will help to make it more understandable as to why the elements found in Himalayan salt are of such benefit to us. Our cells can only absorb what is available to them in either organic or ionic-colloidal form and if the elements aren't available in those forms, then they cannot be absorbed... and what the cell can't absorb can't be metabolized.

Chapter 3: Scientific Studies

Most people these days are understandably skeptical whenever new health advice surfaces and who can blame them?!

The "health lobby" have got it so spectacularly wrong on so many occasions in the past that, to a point, they've lost the trust of the very people they're trying to help and advise.

Remember these?

"Don't eat eggs!"… followed years later with "Eggs are fine and, er, actually they're very good for you."

"Don't eat butter, everybody should have margarine!"… was changed only relatively recently to "Whatever you do, don't eat margarine, it'll kill you. It's much better to eat butter."

"Everybody on skimmed milk!"…changed to "Actually, there are good reasons for drinking full cream milk as it contains good fats that the body needs and has cancer protective properties."

The full English breakfast, after years of vilification and being given the label of "a heart attack on a plate" is now being lauded on many wellbeing websites as one of the healthiest breakfasts you can have!

The list could go on, but you get the idea.

So no wonder the general public are, at best, "cautious" when it comes to new health advice and are looking for proof from properly conducted, independent scientific studies, rather than hearsay, opinion, anecdotal "evidence" and, worst of all, guidelines and advice from politicians… because, of course, they know don't they!

However, various scientific studies have proved what tens of thousands of people have been saying over many, many years; that there are genuine health benefits to be derived from the use of Himalayan salt and salt lamps.

This is by no means the first time that what started out as just opinion has, at a later date, been backed up by science and curiously, how many studies have shown "old wives tales" (or in the current environment of political correctness, should I say, "experienced person's anecdotes"?!) to be based on sound scientific fact?

Remember "eat your greens"? Well, they couldn't have been more correct with their advice, due to the myriad of nutrients and phytochemicals in leafy green vegetables and sprouts.

What about "carrots are good for your eyes"? I think most children just dismissed that phrase as nothing more than a sneaky way to get them to eat the orange stuff! It turns out that Granny was absolutely spot on; the carotenoids in carrots are of <u>immense</u> benefit to eye health, particularly lutein, which is a form of carotenoid that is found in high concentrations within the human eye. In a very recent study, a compound called meso-zeaxanthin has been found to be important to eye health and this substance cannot be found in food sources and appears to be created in the retina from ingested lutein, in other words, from the carrots you eat… so she was right all along!

"An hour before midnight is worth two after it." Well, Granny was right again!

Apparently, major studies on sleep have shown that levels of cortisol and melatonin are dramatically affected not only by how much you sleep, but also, WHEN you sleep, with one study concluding that going to bed late can "fry your hormones, brain, and immune system"... which isn't good news for me, a self-confessed night owl who is desperately trying to reform!

We should have listened to her!

I mention the above because, once again, the positive opinion that many people have had about Himalayan salt has been proved to be well founded by fastidiously conducted scientific studies.

Two significant studies, one in Las Vegas, Nevada, USA in 2007, and one in Austria in 2001, both concluded that significant health benefits can be derived from the use of Himalayan salt.

The 2007 U.S. Study

In this trial, a research lab studied the effects on subjects of drinking a sole made of either Himalayan salt or sea salt on a daily basis and measuring the effects it had upon what is referred to as the Optimum Wellness test. All subjects were in good general health.

The Optimum Wellness test is a system that analyses and evaluates health on a cellular level by way of a 39 point test on urine and saliva.

The subjects were randomly divided up into two groups, one group taking Himalayan salt sole, the other group taking sea salt sole.

Prior to commencement of the study, baseline data was collected by experienced doctors and healthcare professionals from each subject consisting of the following:-

- Optimal Wellness Test via saliva and urine samples
- Heart rate
- Body temperature
- Respiration function
- Blood pressure

The tests were repeated on the 15th day and at the end of the 30-day trial.

The results were grouped into three category zones:-

A Green zone, an Amber zone, and a Red zone for subjects who, upon testing, presented as being up to 5%, up to 15%, and 35% or more respectively away from optimal levels of mineralisation, oxidative stress, and hydration.

At the start of the study, ALL subjects presented in the Red Zone, which, as specified above, is classified as being 35% or more away from an optimum level of wellness as determined by Mineralization, Oxidative Stress, and Hydration.

Every morning for 30 days, each group drank their respective solutions of 1 teaspoon of sole stirred into 237ml of purified water.

The results are shown in table form below:-

All subjects pre-study

	Mineralisation	Oxidative Stress	Hydration
within 5% of optimal	0%	0%	0%
within 15% of optimal	0%	0%	0%
35% or more away from optimal	100%	100%	100%

Sea Salt Group after 30 Days

	Mineralisation	Oxidative Stress	Hydration
within 5% of optimal	0%	4%	6%
within 15% of optimal	16%	19%	13%
35% or more away from optimal	84%	77%	81%

Himalayan Salt Group after 30 Days

	Mineralisation	Oxidative Stress	Hydration
within 5% of optimal	58%	44%	49%
within 15% of optimal	42%	56%	51%
35% or more away from optimal	0%	0%	0%

I think the results shown in the tables above are astonishing! This was a relatively short 30 day trial and when you compare the green and red rows of the pre-study subjects with the same rows of the Himalayan salt study group at the end of the 30-day trial, the difference really is quite remarkable.

The conclusion of the test was that Himalayan salt is highly effective at normalizing mineral levels within the human body, in stabilizing systemic pH and oxidative stress levels, and in helping optimize hydration.

The 2001 Austrian Study

This was an even bigger study that took place at the prestigious Inter-University Graz in Austria, in conjunction with the Institute for Biophysical Research and was conducted over a 9-week period using the internationally recognized double-blind criteria for human research.

At the start of the test, all subjects underwent biophysical and psychological evaluation using the IMEDIS system, which is a biofeedback system created in Russia to monitor the health of Russian cosmonauts while in space. It is still used to this day as an integral part of their space programme.

The participants were then split into 4 groups, each group made up of the same range of subjects in regard to age, weight, sex, and health status.

No other drugs, homeopathic treatments or diets were undertaken during the 9-week study.

Throughout the day, the subjects in each group drank 1.5 liters of either tap water or Fiji water (this is a bottled mineral water originating in Fiji).

The four groups were:-

- Group 1 - Fiji water only
- Group 2 - Tap water only
- Group 3 - Fiji water with 1 teaspoon of Himalayan salt sole solution
- Group 4 - Tap water with 1 teaspoon of common table salt solution

All subjects were re-tested at the end of the trial.

The results of the study were overwhelming and conclusive and to a degree, even surprised the doctors and scientists conducting the trial.

Group 1 and Group 3 both showed a significant positive improvement in organ function, nervous system function, connective tissue status, stomach function, circulatory system, and respiratory function, as well as the kidney and bladder system, the skin, and the spleen and liver system, **with Group 3 subjects showing the best results of all.**

Group 2 and Group 4 both saw a **decline** in the same functions over the nine week period.

Group 3 subjects also showed a decrease in blood pressure and reported an increase in sleep quality, brain activity and concentration levels, energy levels, weight loss, and libido, as well as noticeable nail and hair growth.

As a point of interest, all four groups showed an increase in HDL (High Density Lipoproteins) or "good cholesterol" levels, with the most significant increase coming in Group 1 and Group 2.

The LDL (Low Density Lipoproteins) or "bad cholesterol" levels decreased in all four groups, with the most significant decrease occurring in Group 3 and Group 4.

Medical research has shown that high levels of HDL and low levels of LDL in the blood help against the risk of arteriosclerosis (thickening and hardening of the walls of the arteries).
These tests imply that drinking water throughout the day supports and maintains a higher level of HDL, while a healthy level of salt in our system supports and maintains a healthy, lower level of LDL.

In conclusion, these studies supply us with irrefutable proof as to the benefits of Himalayan salt _from the point of view of its ingestion as 1 teaspoon of an optimally produced sole added to_

1.5 liters of natural spring/mineral water and consumed throughout the day.

I look forward to the day when they conduct the same stringent scientific studies on salt lamps

Chapter 4: The Benefits of Using Himalayan Salt

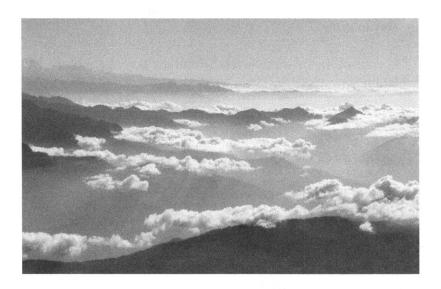

The health benefits derived from the use of Himalayan salt are manyfold. Obviously, everybody's different and as they say, "every body's different" but the majority of the documented positives that come from the use of Himalayan salt are there for all to see and will apply to anyone who is interested in achieving and maintaining optimum health.

I felt that merely compiling a very long list of benefits wouldn't make for a particularly interesting read and, more importantly, there wouldn't be the same opportunity for any "depth" to the important information if it was merely assembled as a bullet point presentation. So I opted to discuss them at varying length, interspersed throughout the book.

As such, it's quite important that the book is read as a whole in order to get the most from it.

That being said, the following is an easy to view list of just <u>some</u> of the health benefits associated with optimal intake levels of Himalayan salt:-

1. The controlling of water levels within the body i.e. water regulation

2. Regulating blood sugar levels

3. Promoting a stable pH balance

4. Aiding in the optimal passing of electric impulses to and from the cells

5. Improving the absorption capabilities of the intestine - meaning that your body is more able to properly absorb the nutrients within the food you consume

6. Supporting a healthy respiratory system, which includes helping alleviate the symptoms of asthma and other COPD type disorders

7. Helping to promote overall vascular health

8. Lowering incidence of sinus problems

9. Promoting greater bone strength

10. Reducing incidents of cramp

11. Improvement in sleep patterns

12. Promoting kidney and gallbladder health

13. Reduction in levels of anxiety and SAD (Seasonal Affective Disorder) symptoms

14. Maintaining a healthy balance of electrolytes within the body, which in turn helps to regulate the heart beat

15. Encouraging the stomach to produce the right amount of hydrochloric acid (HCl) - low levels of HCl are associated with many negative health issues

Himalayan salt also helps in the process of detoxifying the body, particularly from the point of view of eliminating heavy metals from your system (detoxification also takes place by way of the already mentioned balancing of the systemic pH levels).

It also greatly aids in the balancing of hormone levels throughout the body system.

The sodium chloride level of Himalayan salt is lower than that of ordinary table salt and this is obviously a very important factor when considering its health benefits. However, of equal importance is the fact that Himalayan salt has the highest level of potassium than any other salt, including unrefined sea salt.

Many scientific studies have shown that the ratio between sodium and potassium intake is critical, as potassium helps to offset the hypertensive (causing high blood pressure) effects of sodium and although an imbalance of this ratio can lead to hypertension (high blood pressure), it can also be a contributory factor in other diseases like stroke, heart disease, kidney stones, osteoporosis, rheumatoid arthritis, and other ailments.

Himalayan salt contains 0.28% potassium, sea salt contains 0.16%, while table salt contains only 0.09%, and although those numbers represent tiny amounts, the difference is crucial to the body as it can react dramatically to even slight variances in levels and ratios of anything on which it relies.

It is advisable that the reader researches further into the optimal amounts of sodium and potassium intake, as a large 2011 study in the USA showed that those at overall greatest risk of cardiovascular disease were those whose intake was a combination of both too much sodium and too little potassium, with those who ate a lot of salt and very little potassium being twice as likely to die of a heart attack than those who consumed equal amounts of both.

I am NOT implying here that the consumption of Himalayan salt alone will address a possible imbalance of sodium to potassium, as it almost certainly won't. Most people will have to consume other foods like avocados, lima beans, spinach, broccoli, prunes, and other green vegetables to raise their potassium levels to the desired ratio.

The sodium-potassium electrolyte balance ensures proper balance of the fluid in your body's cells, blood plasma, and extracellular fluid.

Another way in which Himalayan salt can aid good health is due to the fact that it can reduce the overall acidity level of the body by way of aiding the excretion of excess acids through urination, thus helping to balance the acid-alkaline ratio. There is a school of thought that suggests a link between higher body acidity levels and Alzheimer's disease.

Mixing two teaspoons of finely ground Himalayan salt with four teaspoons of honey, forming a paste, has been used as a very effective face mask, due to both substances' anti-inflammatory properties. Leave the paste on your skin for 15 minutes (avoiding the eye area), then rinse off with warm water, while at the same time applying gentle circular motions to the skin. It can help calm an outbreak of acne and also hydrates the skin.

Chapter 4: The Benefits of Using Himalayan Salt

People have also used salt to help clear ear infections, either by way of a nasal saline solution to clear any infection of the eustachian tube (which leads to the inner ear), or by using the "salt sock" remedy (I kid you not - this is covered on the highly respected "livestrong.com" website). It basically consists of heating a cup of coarse sea salt/Himalayan salt crystals in a microwave, mix them thoroughly to ensure even temperature distribution throughout the crystals, place the heated crystals in an old sock (!) and being sure that the sock isn't too hot, hold it against the affected ear for 10–15 minutes. They say that this helps control the pain and draws out fluids.

A little known fact about salt in general is that it's crucial for proper adrenal function and the adrenal glands are responsible for the production and regulation of over 50 of the body's hormones.

There is greatly improved mineral status of the entire body and it helps to balance blood pressure, as it provides mineral rich salt in an ionic solution. Due to the magnesium content of Himalayan salt (and sea salt), any unused sodium is quickly eliminated from the body via the kidneys before it can do any harm. Correct quantities of these salts have been shown to equalize or "normalize" blood pressure, lowering it if your blood pressure is too high and raising it to normal if your blood pressure is too low.

Himalayan salts contain selenium which helps to rid the body of toxic heavy metals by attaching to them before expulsion. It also contains boron which is an element that is useful in the prevention of osteoporosis, and chromium, which acts as a regulator of blood sugar levels. It also contains copper, which is used by the body in the maintenance of arterial health.

It is also a powerful antihistamine and antibacterial substance and, furthermore, supports the thyroid and adrenal function.

Because of its antibacterial and antimicrobial properties, the use of Himalayan salt by way of a salt inhaler (please refer to that section of the book) can help purify and detoxify the lungs and sinuses, because the minute salt particles travel through the entire respiratory system, thereby reducing the symptoms of certain lung conditions such as asthma, with some people reporting that after using the salt pipe for a period of time they no longer needed their conventional inhaler (Important:- **NEVER** stop taking prescribed medicines without first having a full consultation with your doctor).

A reduction in seasonal allergies has been widely documented and this is achieved by way of cleansing the sinuses. Congestion and phlegm within the chest is broken down, leading to an improvement in symptoms associated with a heavy cold.

Referring back to point number one on the list, for some people, water retention is a real problem and salt often gets the blame, as indeed it should if they're referring to processed table salt. Himalayan salt does exactly the opposite as it helps the body to properly balance the electrolyte minerals, resulting in the release of any retained water.

Salt water has been used as a mouthwash for centuries. Just add half a teaspoon of salt to half a tumbler of warm water and swill around your mouth before spitting out and rinsing. Due to its antiseptic properties, it eliminates the bacteria that can cause bad breath and gingivitis. Himalayan salt has proved to be particularly effective at this.

Skin conditions such as eczema and dermatitis have been seen to improve with the use of Himalayan salt, either by way of an ingested salt sole, or applied topically.

Remember, consuming too much of ANY kind of salt can result in serious health complications.

However, please take note that studies have shown a possible link between sodium restriction, which leads to a <u>lack</u> of sodium in the body, and insulin resistance (seen in pre or full onset diabetes) and with increased rates of mortality.

In one 4-year-long study involving 100,000 people in 17 different countries, it was found that consuming more than 6 grams of sodium daily raised your risk of health complications, including high blood pressure, BUT, consuming less than 3 grams of sodium per day also led to serious health issues.

It appeared that the optimum daily sodium intake was between 3 and 6 grams, and that while there IS a relationship between sodium intake and blood pressure, this relationship is NOT linear. While consuming more than 6 grams of sodium per day raises your risk of heart disease, so do levels of lower than 3 grams per day.

A famous online doctor once said, "Don't start shoveling salt in your mouth, but <u>do</u> understand the difference between refined table salt and pure, unprocessed salt, which actually serves to support the body, not destroy it. In the right quantities, unrefined salt can be an awesome health promoter."

As with everything in nature, and in particular with the human body, it's a question of striking the right balance.

And as far as Himalayan salt is concerned, it really is a case of:-

Make salt your medicine, not your poison!

Chapter 5: Sea Salt

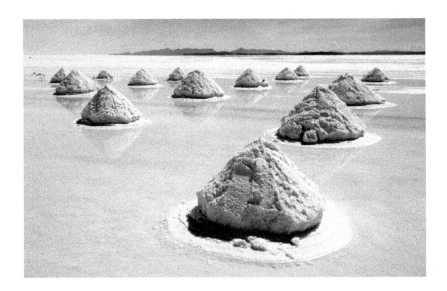

All salts are sea salts in so much as they originate from a salty body of water. It's just that with Himalayan salt and other rock salts, that body of water dried up millions of years ago.

Sea salt is salt that's produced by the evaporation of sea water, as opposed to being mined from sedimentary geological veins. Used extensively in cooking and cosmetics, it's also known as solar salt or bay salt.

There are two main methods of producing commercial sea salt. In one, the technique used is to fill small, interconnected ponds with seawater which is then left to evaporate. The product that is left behind is sea salt. Certain geological and environmental parameters are necessary in order to site the ideal production area of sea salt. The combination of a shallow shoreline, long, hot sunny days, a steady year-round climate, and coastal winds all create the ideal environment for the production and harvesting of sea salt. This why a lot of sea salt is produced along the Mediterranean coast.

Contrary to the popular understanding of the production of sea salt, the solution is moved from container to container, sometimes via gravity and sometimes mechanically, as the concentration of salt within the water alters. The natural salinity of seawater is approximately 3.4%, but by the time this reaches about 25% salinity, the salt will start to crystallize and can then be harvested.

This is actually quite a time intensive process, with some manufacturers claiming that from the point at which the seawater enters the first container, to the point at which the salt is ready to be packed, can take about five years!

Upon reaching the optimal 25% salinity, the crystallised salt can be harvested and then rinsed in brine solution in order to wash out any impurities.

The second method is to pipe salt water into large steel pans. Mud and other impurities will settle to the bottom of the pan as sediment and the remaining water is siphoned off into another pan and heated. As the water heats up, a foam may form on the surface which is skimmed off and the heating of the water continues until it is all evaporated, leaving only the salt crystals behind. Quite often, commercial sea salt manufacturers will add calcium, magnesium, and/or iodide to the salt to provide a characteristic taste and flavour to their particular product.

Using this method, it is obviously of vital importance that the manufacturer sources the seawater from areas of the ocean that are free of pollution, because oil, chemical run-off, and a whole host of other types of pollutants will dramatically affect the quality and taste of the salt.

The colour of the salt is also influenced by the area of the ocean from which the water is taken due to varying ratios of mineral content.

The chemical composition of <u>unrefined</u> sea salt is very similar to that of Himalayan salt, but, as stated previously, those tiny differences in composition make a big difference to the salt's effect on the body. Also, just as with Himalayan salt, the darker the sea salt, the more trace minerals will be present.

However, please be aware that some sea salts can also contain trace amounts of heavy metals due to pollution in the sea water from which they are derived.

Another very important point which may, and indeed should, cause concern, are recent studies (2015-2016) that have found alarming levels of plastic within certain sea salts. They are extremely tiny pieces of plastic, called microplastics, that find their way into the salt on our table, as our oceans continue to fill up with plastic debris and waste, which, in turn, breaks down into smaller and smaller particles of plastic.

Sea birds have been found to have microplastics in their system and plastic debris was present in at least 25% of fish samples taken in Asia and the USA. Some researchers found measurements of more than 1,200 particles of microplastic per 1 lb (0.45 kg) of sea salt.

It's not just that you don't want to be eating plastic! It's the fact that these microplastics are very good at absorbing the pollutants that are in the sea water, and as you ingest them, they deposit these pollutants into your body.

The level of microplastics in the sea salt that was tested is actually less than that found in shellfish, so my advice would be to proceed with caution and definitely to contact the manufacturer of the sea salt that you're considering purchasing

to ask about the quality of the water from which it is derived, with particular regard to possible microplastic contamination.

As far as the chemical composition of sea salt is concerned, the most abundant elements are, as with all salts, sodium and chloride. Chloride in particular helps with muscle and nerve function, while sodium also acts upon muscle function and helps to regulate blood volume and pressure. Sodium is also vitally important in the transmission of signals, both intra-cellular and extra-cellular.

Potassium is an important macromineral (inorganic nutrients that the body requires in large quantities) that, along with chloride, helps to regulate the acid levels within the body.

The ratio of potassium in sea salt is less than that of Himalayan salt, and some experts cite this as the reason why they consider Himalayan salt to be superior.

Sea salt also contains the macrominerals magnesium and calcium, and these play an essential role in several chemical reactions within the body. Magnesium is directly involved in energy production within the cells, and calcium, as is widely known, is essential in the development and maintenance of healthy bones and teeth. In addition, calcium is important for regulating your heartbeat, as well as ensuring normal muscle and nerve function.

The above is also true of Himalayan salt.

The third most abundant element in sea salt, after sodium and chloride, is sulphur. This is not classed as an essential mineral, but plays an important role in the function of your immune system and in general detoxification of the body. Sulphur is the eighth most common element in the human body and it has important roles in normalising metabolism and in helping maintain overall heart health.

Chapter 5: Sea Salt

Just like Himalayan salt, sea salt also contains a good number of trace elements. These include phosphorus, zinc, iron, boron, bromine, manganese, silicon, and copper. The body utilises these trace elements in the production of enzymes that are involved in metabolism. Phosphorus is used in the production of cell membranes and for energy production.

As you can see, there are many similarities between sea salt and Himalayan salt, one of those being that the minerals found in sea salt are present in their natural ratios, and because of this, sea salt also helps keep the body's electrolytes in balance.

Many of the various sea salts are produced in such a way that the end product has larger sized individual crystals, which means that you can use less salt to season food and get the same effect. The outcome is that you can actually reduce your sodium intake while still enjoying the "kick" from a larger size salt crystal. Table salt is normally ground to a very fine powder and, as such, cannot achieve this "pop" on the tongue.

Although this is a book primarily about Himalayan salt and its derivative products, it is a fact that a lot of chefs, culinary experts, and "foodies" prefer the taste and texture of sea salt above that of Himalayan salt. I think this is less to do with the slightly different mineral ratios and more to do with the fabulous pop or "explosion" of taste on the tongue that you can get from the larger crystals which are very often a characteristic of sea salt.

Just as with Himalayan salt, unrefined sea salt also helps the kidneys to rid the body of excess acidity, while also aiding in the regulation of blood sugar levels.

The iodine content of sea salt is relatively high and this enables the thyroid gland to manufacture the necessary hormones required for optimal body functioning, growth, and development.

In conclusion, both Himalayan salt and sea salts are referred to as "full spectrum" salts, with the inherent complete range of trace elements and minerals remaining intact. However, it's important to make sure when purchasing sea salt that it is pure, unrefined sea salt.

Not all sea salts are created equally and it's easy to be misled by packaging that looks impressive and appears to say all the right things, when actually the product inside is merely a variation of table salt, having undergone the same intense heat treatment that strips away 82 of the 84 naturally occurring elements and minerals. It <u>must</u> say "unrefined" or "unprocessed" on the packaging.

Genuine sea salt is slightly moist, usually of larger crystal size, and a little more towards a grey colour.

If the salt is pure white and powder dry, the alarm bells should start ringing... <u>however</u>, it must be said that some pure sea salt manufacturers do finely grind the salt for customer convenience, but in doing this you may lose a little of the "pop" on the tongue, and you may have to add a few grains of rice to the salt shaker in order to stop clumping, due to the moist nature of pure sea salt.

So, sea salt is a fabulous product and a million times better than ordinary table salt, with a good number of culinary experts preferring it to Himalayan salt for its use in cooking, **but just make sure it's unrefined sea salt**... and don't forget to enquire about the quality of the sea water from which it is made.

Celtic Sea Salt is harvested in a way that appeals to my instinctive lean towards natural production methods. It is harvested from Atlantic sea water off the coast of Brittany, France. The sea water collects in clay ponds and is allowed to evaporate naturally by way of the sun and air only (no artificial heating) and is gathered using wooden rakes so that no metal touches the salt. That's it... nothing added, nothing taken away. A real quality product.

Chapter 5: Sea Salt

Although this isn't to do with sea salt as such, I want to mention the following from an environmental point of view.

If you're reading this book in the United States and are concerned about the carbon footprint that might be associated with the importation of salts from Asia or Europe, then I encourage you to fully research the "home produced" salts from the US, as long as you're certain to check out the mineral analysis of each product to make sure that the health promoting elements are present and to the optimal ratios.

Redmond Real Salt looks like an amazing product. Made from salt deposits from a sea that used to cover a large area of North America millions of years ago, it is an unrefined, unprocessed, unpolluted salt from an ancient sea, with all the minerals and inherent flavour left intact. (They've also invested in solar panels at their Utah location, to the extent that almost all of the operations at the site are now powered by solar energy... which very much ticks the environmental box for me).

Purchasing an unrefined, top quality, locally produced salt can have real environmental advantages for those living in the US.

The same principle applies for the UK, although it has to be said that *Celtic Sea Salt*, being manufactured in Brittany, France, isn't exactly a million miles away.
However, there are three manufacturers that are worthy of mention, as all three claim that their product and manufacturing processes retain the high levels of trace elements worthy of a quality salt. Those companies are *Maldon Salt* based in Essex, *Cornish Sea Salt*, and *Halen Mon* based in Wales, although I'm sure there will be more.

I must emphasize that, personally, I think it's more important to put the health benefits derived from the use of a quality, unrefined salt from further afield above any possible environmental consequences of not sourcing locally.

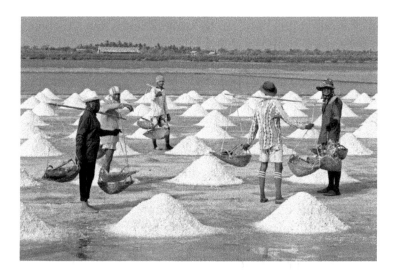

Harvesting salt from the sea

Chapter 6: Iodized Salt

Iodine is a non-metallic mineral that the body requires in only trace amounts, but nonetheless, an iodine deficiency can lead to many health complications, including weight gain, slowed metabolism, and intolerance to cold, as well as gastrointestinal and neurological abnormalities. It is vital for pregnant and nursing mothers to make sure that they are taking in an optimal amount of iodine, as its deficiency can impede foetal and newborn development, with iodine deficiency being the most common cause of preventable brain damage in children the world over.

Iodized salt was introduced into the United States in 1924 in an effort to halt the ever-rising number of goitre cases (a goitre being a swelling of the neck caused by an enlarged thyroid gland). The greatest concentration of iodine is to be found in the thyroid gland.

Health problems arising from iodine deficiency are still prevalent in certain parts of South America, central Asia, and Africa. Iodine is available naturally through the consumption of, amongst others, salt water fish and other seafood, kelp, and vegetables grown in iodine rich soils.

From 1924, wind the clock forward to 1995 when the World Health Assembly (WHA) decided to adopt universal salt iodization, which meant that all salt for human and livestock consumption needed to be iodized. This was to help eliminate iodine deficiency disease, such as myxoedema, cretinism, and neurological disorders in children, as well as those listed above. Due to the WHA resolution, countries throughout the world routinely require iodine to be added to salt.

However, the inherent problem with this philosophy is that iodizing table salt is a very crude form of prevention and is likely to only be necessary for those people living under the desperate conditions of famine. People in more developed countries who are fortunate enough to enjoy a relatively well-balanced diet are not at risk of iodine deficiency, due to the fact that there are appropriate levels of iodine in many food sources, including the aforementioned sea fish and shell fish, as well as cereal grains, eggs, legumes, and dairy products, as the cows themselves will have been fed a diet that incorporated iodized salt.

And for those that might say, "Hey, I know they've stripped all the good stuff from the salt, but look, they've added iodine" is a bit like saying to someone, "Hey, I know they've just taken $10,000 from your bank account, but look, they've given you $5 back".

It is possible, particularly in the West and all developed countries, to take in too much iodine, resulting in an iodine overload. Up to 75% of iodine within the body is stored in the thyroid gland, which itself is involved in the production of hormones that regulate body metabolism, and in just the same way that too little iodine can cause many health problems, then too much iodine can cause the production of these hormones to become dangerously unbalanced, which can lead to metabolic issues and immune disorders. Too much iodine can also lead to an increased heart rate and high blood pressure, hand tremors, abnormal heart rhythms, as well as anxiety and general nervousness.

So, in conclusion, although iodine is a very important constituent of the diet, unless you live in a part of the world where you don't have access to a varied diet, you don't need to rely on salt that has been iodized in order to achieve the necessary levels.

Chapter 7: Himalayan Bath Salts

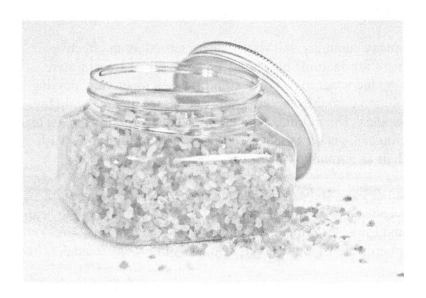

Most of us have taken the time out to enjoy relaxing in a nice, hot bath after a hard day at work. It really is one of life's little pleasures!

Salt baths are relaxing, detoxifying and rejuvenating, and there's something about the stillness, silence and being at peace that leads to a feeling of deep relaxation, and has been proved to reduce tension and help regulate stress hormones.

Of course, there's nothing new about the use of salts in baths - the Ancient Greeks were using them thousands of years ago, as did the Egyptians and Romans. In the UK, whole towns were built around the rising popularity of health spas, hence towns with names like "Leamington Spa" and "Bath" became famous for their rejuvenative waters.

As a point of interest, the term for the medical use of sea water/salt water as a therapy to treat various ailments is thalassotherapy, from the Greek word thalassa, meaning "sea".

Over many centuries, salt water has been used as an effective treatment for dandruff by adding 3 tbsp of salt to warm water, allowing the water to cool to a comfortable temperature, pouring the solution onto the hair and scalp, and massaging the scalp for 6-7 minutes. This is quite a long time to have your arms in the air, so if you can, get somebody else to massage it in for you. Wash your hair as normal to finish.

Salt water has also been used to aid in the treatment of spots, acne and eczema, and of course, the old paddle on the seashore to heal foot and lower leg wounds/infections is legendary, as is fishermen's use of sea water to help heal almost any wound.

The treatment of disease by bathing in mineral-rich water is known as balneotherapy, and, as you've read, Himalayan salts have been used for many years as a safe and effective way to relax and help heal the body, especially when it comes to healing the skin.

Salt water has been shown to help alleviate the symptoms of psoriasis (a skin disease characterized by red, itchy, scaly patches) because of its antiseptic qualities, and because it leads to better skin hydration.

When you take a salt bath, the salt forms an ionic solution and minerals such as potassium, sodium, zinc, iodine, copper, iron, calcium, manganese, and magnesium are absorbed through the skin as ions in a process known as "dermal absorption".

This process means that having a salt water bath with Himalayan salts may help with:

- Insect bites and nettle stings
- Wounds and blisters
- A recurring skin infection that is not responding to treatment
- Gynecological hygiene
- As part of your care regimen after having surgery
- Joint pain - including rheumatism
- Some people have reported a reduction in cellulite (although the author has seen no evidence supporting this claim)
- Various skin conditions
- Relaxing cramped muscles (great for if you've been hitting the gym!)
- Relief of certain respiratory conditions and sinus infections (achieved by way of the inhalation of the steam from the salt water)

Something that you may find interesting is that the bath water is going to remain at a more constant temperature when using Himalayan salt. This is because the biophysical composition of the salt is such that the molecules continue moving in a constant rhythm for some time.

Getting the most out of a Himalayan salt bath

Simply run a bath to the level and temperature of your choice (though studies show the optimum water temperature to be just about body temperature – 37 C or 97 F) and add 2 cups of Himalayan salt. If you wish to be a little more precise in your measurements, then 2.5lbs (1.1kgs) of salt per average size bath is optimal.

(If you just want to use your salt bath to soothe your skin, then adding only 1/3lb (0.15kgs) to the water is sufficient).

When using these kinds of salts, make sure that you don't add anything else to the water. Oils, soaps, and other bath additives can reduce the effectiveness of the salts. You should bathe for at least 20 - 30 minutes in order to fully benefit from their effect.

As well as the minerals listed above being absorbed into the body, when you have a salt bath, some toxins will exit the body by way of a process called "reverse osmosis".

A 2010 study found that soaking in a saline solution, like a salt water bath, may help to reduce the inflammation associated with arthritis, rheumatism, and similar inflammatory conditions.

After having soaked in a salt bath for a period of time, there is contradictory advice as to the next phase of the bathing process. Some experts advocate finishing off with a shower in order to wash away any recently exited toxins that may be on the surface of the skin, while others recommend not showering and to merely gently pat yourself dry, so as not to remove any remaining salt from the skin in order that it may continue to do its work for longer.

Obviously, this decision is entirely that of the individual, as both methodologies make sense.

It's usually a good idea to drink moderate amounts of fluids while taking a warm water salt bath, as this will keep you hydrated.

If you ever feel slightly dizzy or in any way a little unwell while having a salt bath, it is recommended that you carefully get out of the bath to cool off, sit quietly and have a drink of water.

Not only does the electrical charge of the salt within the water, in conjunction with the dissolved minerals, detoxify and deep cleanse the skin, but also the magnesium and other trace minerals help to heal damaged or cramped muscles and other soft tissue and connective structures.

It's worth noting that having a bath using normal water with no added salt will actually pull or extract moisture and salt from the skin, because body fluids are themselves a saline/salt solution, so the two entities (i.e. your body and the bath water) will try to achieve a state of equilibrium. This process results in the tell-tale wrinkly skin that we've probably all noticed sometimes. This doesn't happen when you have a salt bath, because water and minerals are actually absorbed into the skin.

To add to the experience, it can really help if you're able to dim the lights, and for some people, have relaxing, soothing music playing, although others prefer the solitude of absolute silence.

Beeswax candles are very effective too, but please DON'T use ordinary petroleum based tee lights, as they give off more toxic air pollutants than if you had somebody in the bathroom with you smoking a cigarette!

It's a good idea to take the opportunity to meditate a little and engage in some mindfulness to take you into an even deeper state of relaxation.

I would also strongly recommend at some point while bathing engaging in a spot of yogic breathing. In itself, this type of breathing has been shown to reap a myriad of health benefits, but coupled with the relaxing effect of the warm water, its therapeutic action is even more powerful.

Simply put, yogic breathing is the practice of breathing from the diaphragm. If you were to put one hand on your stomach, and the other hand on your chest, as you breathe in through the nose, the hand on your stomach should be pushed outwards, while the hand on your chest should remain relatively still. This is known as "diaphragmatic breathing" and it ensures that the lungs fill to full capacity from the bottom upwards.

The action is not forced and the shoulders should remain loose and down throughout, not rising up to your ears. You should breathe out through your mouth, again not forcing and not allowing the chest to collapse. All the movement, both in and out, should come from the diaphragm. This is not necessarily deep breathing, as there's a difference between yogic breathing and deep breathing. Yogic breathing should remain relaxed, easy, and unforced at all times.

The benefits that can be gained from this simple but effective breathing practice are tremendous and I certainly encourage all readers to further research this subject - I'm sure you won't regret it!

As far as your warm, relaxing bath is concerned, I can guarantee you will feel great afterwards, your skin will feel clean and refreshed, and it will probably be the first of many times you'll enjoy this little bit of pampering.

You can use Real Salt, Celtic Salt, or most unrefined sea salts to experience similar benefits, but probably at a lower price.

So, all of the above health benefits, both physical and emotional, can be derived just from having a simple salt water bath.

Not bad for just lying in lovely warm water!

Please note - *Because of the extra strain put on the circulatory system, people with diabetes, any heart condition, kidney disease, blood pressure issues (high OR low), liver disease, any circulatory issues, and pregnant women should **ALL** consult with a qualified health practitioner before taking a salt bath.*

Chapter 8: Himalayan Salt Inhalers (Salt Pipes)

Salt air therapy, also referred to as "speleotherapy", is the practice of inhaling salt-laden air and if you're looking for the most convenient method by which to benefit from salt air therapy, then a salt inhaler is probably the best option.

If you've ever seen someone use an inhaler for their allergies or their asthma, then the idea behind the salt inhaler is exactly the same, in that you use the inhaler to administer the salts via direct inhalation.

Hippocrates, who is considered the father of modern medicine (hence the Hippocratic oath), used to administer a treatment of steaming salt to help his patients achieve full and proper lung function.

When using the salt pipe, you place the mouthpiece between your lips, inhale through the mouth and then exhale through the nose, which is actually the opposite of normal breathing. As you breathe in, air is sucked in through the bottom of the device, passes through the salt in the middle chamber and continues its journey through your mouth and into the lungs.

The warm, moist air of the breath absorbs microscopic particles of salt ions which are rapidly absorbed into the lungs. The salt gets to work on any mucus that may be lining the bronchial passages and in the bronchial sacs of the lungs themselves (which is a common symptom of many pulmonary disorders) by breaking down the mucus, and due to its anti-inflammatory and anti-bacterial effects, also immediately starts to calm down any inflammation. This can help with many common ailments,

Himalayan Salt and Himalayan Salt Lamps

including congestion, hay fever, allergies, chest infections, asthma, flu, and even the common cold.

Unlike other inhalers, such as those used to administer pharmaceutical drugs or steroid inhalers, this approach is completely safe and will not result in any of the negative side effects or contraindications that are often associated with other therapies.

Rather, these inhalers are easy to use, will help you to avoid many common respiratory conditions, come with no side effects, and as such are a treatment that anyone can use.

A very famous TV doctor in the UK discussed these inhalers on a networked morning show and spoke very highly of them, saying that his own secretary used them to help relieve her asthma and that one of his patients had stopped using her regular prescription asthma inhaler altogether since starting to use the salt pipe! He went on to say that all she did was use the salt pipe for about 10 minutes per day while watching her favourite TV show. It didn't take any time out of her day and she was able to ditch the drugs - now there's a win-win situation!

Obviously, NEVER stop taking medicines prescribed by your doctor without first consulting them.

The benefits of using a salt pipe/salt inhaler are numerous and they include:

- Helping with sinus ailments - if you have trouble with your sinuses or want to bolster up the overall strength of your lungs and respiratory system, you should use a salt inhaler. There are some studies found from the 1800s that show breathing in salt air, or the salt that came from mines, was a great way to reduce some common respiratory problems and could help alleviate irritation caused by air pollution.

- Supports the cleansing of harmful organisms - it is not uncommon for such organisms to find their way into your lungs. Salt inhalers are able to help safely "clean up" harmful bacteria (salt is a natural anti-bacterial agent).

- Detoxifies the air - no matter where you live, there are probably issues with air quality. You may live with a smoker, or you live in an area where air pollution is very high. Few of us live near the ocean (or in a salt mine!) so aren't able to reap the benefits of such locations, but a salt inhaler can give welcome relief from dust, smoke, pet dander, smog, and other airborne pollutants.

- Lower blood pressure - there are some studies that show that the potassium absorbed via the use of a salt inhaler is effective in helping to stabilize blood pressure. If you are suffering from high blood pressure, it may be worth consideration, *but obviously ONLY if approved by your medical practitioner/GP/health care professional after discussing it with them during a consultation.*

- Promotes mental calmness - there are times when your breathing is going to become laboured because you are upset, anxious or stressed. A salt inhaler helps by encouraging you to take deeper and longer breaths, resulting in a calmer and more controlled state of mind.

- Helps you get a good night's sleep - salt pipe inhalers help balance the histamine response (an immune system response to foreign pathogens) of the lungs, sinuses, and bronchial tract, and so reduce the symptoms of night coughs, breath related sleeping conditions, and snoring that may keep you up at night, or make it difficult to get into a deep and sound sleep.
Poor quality of sleep can have a very serious effect upon your overall health, as sleep deprivation can cause untold damage to your hormone levels and immune system, so

you end up in a vicious cycle of health problems (the author <u>strongly</u> advises the reader to make further studies in connection with sleep deprivation in general, as it is a much misunderstood and relatively little known cause of more health problems than may be realized).

- Moisturizes the mucus membranes.
- It has been used to improve overall lung capacity (this is of benefit to everybody, but can be of considerable importance if you are a singer, brass instrument player or an athlete of any kind).
- Developing the ability to breathe deeply promotes the body's natural relaxation response and auto-immune system, as has been shown over thousands of years via the practice of yogic breathing.
- As salt is a natural expectorant, it can help in reducing the production of excess mucus in the nose (if you're brave enough, you could try a Netti pot, whereby you pour lukewarm/body temperature salt solution into your nasal cavities to clear them of mucus and bacteria).

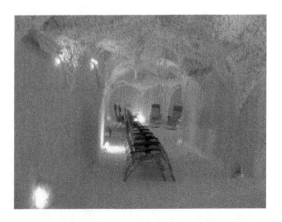

A salt cave used for speleotherapy

Chapter 8: Himalayan Salt Inhalers (Saltpipes)

Some people would be surprised to learn that there is nothing new about the use of salt inhalation therapy. It dates back to the ancient Greeks, but most interestingly, its benefits were noted in Poland in the 18th century.

Polish salt miners were renowned for their good health and strong immune systems and they usually had better health than most of their families, and in a time when lung ailments were commonplace, the Polish salt miners were relatively free of respiratory problems.

On the rare occasions when they did succumb to a cold, the symptoms were usually very mild and the recovery time was swift. All of this at the time, which has since been proved, was attributed to the daily inhalation of salt particles.

A day out at the seaside is an occasion that countless people have enjoyed over hundreds of years. People love to stand on the promenade or on the beach and breathe in the sea air, which is, of course, heavy with salt. People have always found this invigorating and rejuvenating.

If the ocean is too far away, you may be able to benefit from the many salt rooms that are popping up around the world, like the ones to be found in London and New York. These rooms emulate European salt caves and provide an opportunity to help people from densely populated and heavily polluted areas who may be suffering with breathing difficulties to "detoxify" and clear their airways.

However, you don't have to take a trip to the coast or sit in a salt room to benefit from salt inhalation, as you can simply use a salt inhaler. Not only does this actually work extremely well, but one of the beauties of this type of therapy is that it's a small device that's easy to operate and you can use it while you're watching television, listening to the radio, reading a book or browsing the internet. Or just sit back for 15-20 minutes of "me" time and relax, listening to some peaceful music while using the salt inhaler. A great way to unwind, clear your airways, and as a lot of people report, clear their minds as well.

If you, or someone you know, suffers from any chronic respiratory ailments such as sinusitis, asthma, bronchitis or any other COPD (Chronic Obstructive Pulmonary Disease), then I would certainly recommend the use of salt pipes, ***after consultation and confirmation from your doctor.***

If they work for you, as indeed they do for many people, then you could reduce your reliance on drug-based inhalers or other steroidal medication. The theory behind the salt pipe is that it emulates the effect of speleotherapy, in so much that the air you breathe in when using a salt pipe is very similar in composition to the air in a natural salt cave. Also, it is very small and light and can be placed in a handbag or briefcase and taken anywhere, so you reap all the respiratory benefits of a salt cave in the comfort of your own home. (The author would recommend and prefers the use of ceramic salt pipes as it is a more natural container for the delivery of a completely natural product. However, the plastic versions have the advantage of being less likely to break in transit).

As mentioned, the breathing technique to be employed while using a salt inhaler is that of breathing in through the mouth and out through the nose. For people who practice yogic breathing, as more and more people are, this may seem counterintuitive, as they have been encouraged to breathe in through the nose and out through the mouth. However, the principle of filling your lungs from the bottom upwards, as used in yogic breathing or qigong breathing, remains the same, which is as follows:-

Breathing technique while using the salt pipe

Breathing in through your mouth, fill your lungs from the bottom, to the middle, to the top, hold for a second or so and then gently breathe out through your nose, emptying the lungs from the top to the bottom.

It is bad practice to exhale through your mouth while the salt pipe is still in place.

There should be no forced breathing, everything should be relaxed and gentle, but deep.

Continue doing this for 10-15 minutes, preferably on a daily basis.

The above breathing technique in itself has a calming effect and is used in many meditative practices. This alone can help bring your breathing under control if, as the author fully understands from personal experience, you are starting to feel anxious about your shallow breathing and the possible onset of an asthma attack.

Please remember though, if you're not using the salt pipe, you should always breathe in through the nose and out through the mouth for optimal wellbeing.

Maintenance of the salt pipe couldn't be easier, as to clean it you simply wash it with warm water and soap and replace the crystals as and when needed just as you would when replacing salt in a salt cellar, always using large, coarse Himalayan salt crystals. Just remove the stopper and replenish.

According to research, the amount of salt taken in when using a salt pipe is tiny and represents only the merest fraction of what is in or on the food we eat and, as such, has no effect on blood pressure. This tiny amount, however, is so effective because it is going exactly where it is needed.

As said, it is recommended that you use the salt inhaler for between 10 and 15 minutes per day, but this can be split up into 2 or 3 lots of 5 minute sessions spread throughout the day if that's more convenient.

There is an argument for dividing the speleotherapy sessions up anyway, as three separate sessions taken at intervals throughout the day might be of greater overall benefit than one long session, but there is, as yet, no hard evidence as to whether or not this is the case. One way or another, you will reap the benefits.

There are no known or reported side effects from the use of salt pipes, and it is an affordable, convenient, effective, 100% natural treatment.

Additional information:-

Just prior to publication, I came across a magazine article entitled "Salty Yoga". This is a new exercise craze coming out of New York in which yoga is performed in a room where the floor and walls are covered in salt. As you perform the yoga poses, you are encouraged to breathe slowly and deeply, and in doing so, take in microscopic particles of airborne salt. I think this is a great idea as it combines the indisputable physical, mental, and emotional benefits that you get from the practice of yoga, along with the previously discussed health benefits of breathing salty air.

I really fancy giving this a go!

Chapter 8: Himalayan Salt Inhalers (Saltpipes)

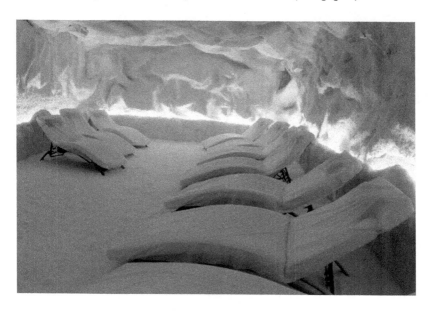

Halotherapy section of a salt cave in Spain

Chapter 9: Himalayan Salt Water (Sole)

More and more people are experiencing the benefits of sole water (pronounced solay). This is a mixture of mineral rich, unrefined salt and water.

The word "sole" comes either from the Latin "sol" meaning sun, or is of Germanic influence from the German word for brine, although the true origin of the word is up for debate!

To some, the idea of drinking salt water may seem counterintuitive, but as long as the salt solution is made using unprocessed natural salt, like Himalayan salt or unrefined sea salt, then it can be of immense benefit to the body.

Salt water is extremely important in the process of digestion, as right from the moment food enters the mouth, it activates the salivary glands, thus releasing the enzyme amylase, which helps digest carbohydrates. In the stomach, natural salts, including Himalayan salt, stimulate the production of hydrochloric acid, which helps to break down food.
This is such an important part of the digestive process, as hydrochloric acid also kills harmful pathogens and bacteria and makes it easier for proteins to be digested. If undigested food accumulates in the stomach, it will result in heartburn and acid reflux, as the food will begin to ferment and produce excess gases.

The drinking of warm, natural salt water actually supports the stomach's function. It also stimulates secretions in the intestinal tract and from the liver, both of which are processes that increase nutrient absorption.

Sole salt water solution also helps reduce inflammation. The body's requirement of salt is no more than 6g per day, which is around one teaspoon, and if we don't consume this amount, the body can enter what is called "crisis mode", which can have, as you can probably guess from the term, considerably negative consequences. If we don't take in enough salt, then the levels of the enzyme renin, and the hormone aldosterone, will rise rapidly. If this rise is maintained over a period of time, it can lead to circulatory damage and increased inflammation within the body. Research has shown that prolonged lack of salt can lead to an increased risk of numerous chronic diseases, including cardiovascular disease and cognition loss.

It has been established that natural salt has a unique effect on stress levels. In an article published in the Journal of Neuroscience, they showed how salt helps alleviate anxiety and that it can raise your oxytocin levels.
Oxytocin is a hormone that helps put you in a more relaxed state of being, so it could be a good idea to raise your oxytocin levels prior to bed by drinking your salt water approximately an hour before sleep.

Salt solution also helps with the detoxification process because of its antibacterial properties. Warm, natural salt water is designed to flush out waste and toxins by simultaneously cleansing the digestive tract and stimulating bowel movement.

Mineral balance within the body is of vital importance, to the extent that some physicians state that you can trace every sickness, every disease, and every ailment to a mineral deficiency. Every system in the body needs minerals to work properly and that includes the production of amino acids and enzymes. Mineral deficiencies are becoming more and more commonplace, however, sole made with natural Himalayan salt is a very good source of all the natural vitamins and trace elements your body needs.

Studies of people using appropriate quantities of salt water have
shown that the participants experienced desired weight loss,
reduced blood pressure, reduced blood sugar, and improved
energy levels.

How to make sole salt water

1. Using a Mason jar, add unrefined Himalayan salt crystals until
the jar is 1/3 full.

2. Add filtered or spring water leaving a 2 inch (5cm) space at
the top.

3. Cover this solution with a glass cap/lid (the lid can be wooden
or plastic if absolutely necessary, but **mustn't** be metal, as the
metal will react with the salt water).

4. Stir or shake the solution and let it stand for 24 hours.

5. If all the salt crystals have dissolved after 24 hours, add a little
more salt.

6. Continue adding small amounts of salt crystals until you can
no longer add any more (i.e. no more salt will dissolve and there
are undissolved salt crystals visible at the bottom of the jar. This
is the obvious sign that the solution is saturated and no more salt
can be dissolved).

As long as it's kept properly covered, the salt water solution will
last indefinitely due to its antibacterial and antifungal properties.

How to take salt water

Every day, to a glass of warm or cold filtered/spring water, add between half and one teaspoon of sole solution, and drink.

This amount will provide you with approximately 240mg to 480mg (half a teaspoon to one full teaspoon respectively) of sodium, which is 10-20%, again respectively, of the RDA (Recommended Daily Allowance) of sodium intake.

Some people prefer to add one teaspoon of sole to 1.5 liters of water in a drinking flask, so that they can take it with them and drink the water at intervals throughout the day.

As a footnote, research has proved that the ancestral diet had salt consumption of between 1.5 and 3 tablespoons (tablespoons!) per day. This level coincided with the lowest risk of heart disease, but of course that will have been using natural, unrefined salt.

Salt is an ionic compound which means that it will completely dissociate when it's dissolved and form an electrolyte solution. When salt (NaCl) is dissolved in water, the resulting solution does not contain complete molecules of NaCl, but rather, it contains the ions of Na+ and Cl-. *It is these ions that the body needs and indeed craves, and is why a sole is of such benefit to our health and wellbeing.*

OK, so salt is an electrolyte, but what exactly does that mean?

The dictionary definition of an electrolyte in solution is:-

"Physiology - Any of various ions, such as potassium, sodium, or chloride (recognize those?!), *required by cells to regulate the electric charge and flow of water across the cell membrane".*

Pretty important stuff this sole!

Your body is a complex and very finely balanced mechanism of cells, tissues, organs, and fluids which, every second of every day, are governed by an almost unimaginable array of precisely orchestrated electrical impulses. The systems only function properly because all those cells, tissues and surrounding fluids exist in a homeostatic environment where electricity is conducted in an efficient way to carry the various signals to their intended destinations.

The key to maintaining this delicate homeostatic environment is through electrolytes.

When electrolytes such as salt dissolve in water, they break apart into their constituent ions, thus creating an electrically conductive solution. Any solution that conducts electricity, such as a salt sole, is therefore known as an electrolyte solution.

Within the human body are several common electrolytes which serve very specific functions, but most of these are, in one way or another, responsible for maintaining the proper balance of fluids between the intracellular environment (inside the cell) and extracellular environment (outside the cell). Like most things in the body, an adequate balance is critical to the proper functioning of the systems. Too much or too little of any electrolyte, creating what's called an electrolyte imbalance, is detrimental to overall health. However, this balance is naturally maintained through proper nutrition and fluid intake.

The six major electrolytes within the human body are:-

1. Sodium (Na)
2. Chloride (Cl)
3. Potassium (K)

4. Magnesium (Mg)
5. Calcium (Ca)
6. Phosphate (PO4)

It will probably be of no surprise to learn that Himalayan salt contains <u>all six</u> of the major electrolytes!

When we drink an electrolyte solution like the many sports drinks that are available - the whole concept of which is based on quick and efficient hydration because they contain one or more electrolytes - and, as is the case in discussion, a salt water sole, we are taking in an electrically charged solution filled with the necessary minerals, macrominerals, trace elements, and electrolytes that help the body maintain a proper pH balance and an optimum electrolyte composition in the fluids that are both part of and surrounding every cell of the body.

A healthy pH balance within the body is a greatly underestimated and under-discussed health topic and a misunderstanding of its importance can lead to all kinds of health problems, which can include reduction in bone density, development of kidney stones, and immune system issues.

Testing your body's pH level couldn't be easier as you can simply take a saliva test. Ideally, this should show a reading of between 6.5 and 7.5, with the vast majority of people who present with a pH imbalance leaning towards the more acidic side, that is, lower than 6.5.
Because salt water is slightly alkaline, this imbalance has been seen to be easily corrected by drinking salt solution or a sole, preferably made with Himalayan salt.

There is anecdotal support for the theory that, because of its positive effects upon the circulatory system, Himalayan salt can be of benefit to people who suffer with chilled extremities, such as is the case with the somewhat unpleasant symptoms associated with Raynaud's disease. (The author must point out that he personally hasn't seen any evidence to support this claim, but feels that there is nothing to lose and everything to gain by at least trying sole therapy as a way of helping to ease this potentially unpleasant condition).

The body absorbs electrolytes faster than it can absorb water alone, but when the two are combined, the body takes in the resulting solution, thereby hydrating much faster.

This is the principle behind "Ionic" or "Hydrating" commercial sports soft drinks which contain the same hydrating minerals as a salt water drink, but with one major downside... they usually also contain ladles of sugar or, worse still, artificial sweeteners such as aspartame and other chemical nasties you really don't want if you're trying to stay healthy!

I regularly have a glass of sole solution in warm water in the morning instead of the usual cup of tea or coffee. It's not something I endure for the sake of my health, it's a pleasurable way to start the day. It tastes fresh and has a little "edge" to it, as opposed to the more "dulling" alternatives.

Drinking the salt water sole also helps your body to hydrate efficiently and to the right levels, without becoming too dilute. We have entered an era where people in the developed world are being encouraged to drink a lot of water. I'm sure you've seen many people walking around with their bottles of mineral water in hand or having it placed strategically on their desk at school or at work. It has got to the point where we are in danger of accidentally <u>over drinking</u>. There is now a body of evidence advocating that you only drink when you are thirsty.

It's funny how everything seems to come back round to doing things naturally. Eat when you're hungry, drink when you're thirsty, and make sure that what you eat and drink is natural, unprocessed, and unrefined, with nothing added or taken away.

It is said that, obviously depending on body size and certain other factors, that the minimum amount of water that you should drink each day is 2 litres (3.52 pints). If you aren't using a sole solution, for each litre (1.76 pints), stir in 1/8 of a teaspoon of Himalayan salt, drink and over the days and weeks, start to feel the difference.

And no, drinking this will NOT make you thirsty (as I used to think it would!), because using Himalayan salt (or unrefined sea salt) actually hydrates the body, due to its balancing effect upon the electrolyte levels.

So, organic natural foods eaten when you're hungry, and natural, unadulterated water (from a glass bottle) drunk when you're thirsty, is the best way forward. Your own body is your best teacher, and will tell you when you're hungry or thirsty. And the little sprinkling of natural Himalayan pink salt on your food or in your water, with its 84 trace elements, minerals, and electrolytes, will be of great benefit.

Drinking water with a little bit of salt as a salt sole means your body will only absorb the amount of fluid that it needs. When we drink water for the sake of drinking, and in particular if the water contains no salt, it tends to be excreted very shortly afterwards, as the body desperately tries to maintain the proper balance between minerals and water. People who permanently walk around with a bottle of water in their hands are usually the same ones who are constantly going to the toilet!

If you are one of the many people who suffer from having to get up and use the bathroom at least once during the night, drinking the sole could be of great benefit, as it will help your body maintain the proper ratio of fluid to minerals and can help prevent the need to urinate during the night.

As far as actual salt consumption is concerned, there have been many studies recently refuting the long held belief that the level of salt intake is linearly correlated to blood pressure levels. For a good few years now, certain sections of the scientific community have been uncomfortable with the advice being given to the public in connection with higher levels of salt intake and a possible/probable rise in blood pressure.

The problem is that just when one study shows there might not be as strong a connection as previously thought, along comes another study to show that there IS a definite connection between salt intake and blood pressure. No one side has definitively won the debate, and the opinions and arguments, both for and against, look set to run for a good while longer yet!

This is a book all about Himalayan salt and Himalayan salt lamps, and I would never profess to be an expert about the causes of high blood pressure by any stretch of the imagination, and because blood pressure is such a vitally important subject of potentially life-ending or life-changing proportions, I strongly encourage the reader to embark on further research into salt intake and possible relative health issues, like heart disease, high blood pressure, and strokes, to find the evidence for themselves and to make an informed decision, but most definitely while also consulting with their personal health care professional.

Also, many people have reported an improvement in blood sugar levels after using a salt sole.

It can be a powerful, natural antihistamine due to its natural balancing effect upon the body.

For centuries, people have gargled with salt water to help clear throat infections, or swilled their mouths to help heal gum disease.

Sole also helps maintain bone density, as the body uses calcium stored in the bones to neutralise any acidity of the blood. Sole is an alkaline and naturally balances the blood pH levels, which means that the body no longer needs to leech calcium from the bones.

It has also been reported that drinking salt water sole can aid weight loss and it is thought this is achieved by the sole improving full and proper digestion and aiding the body in maintaining a proper mineral balance on a cellular level.

Improvement in skin, hair, and nails is also widely reported by the use of a daily salt solution and this is due to the high mineral content of Himalayan salt.

A factor overlooked by most people is the amount of water that we lose during sleep. Significant amounts are lost through respiration and perspiration. Fully hydrating first thing in the morning is a practice which can be of huge benefit to your body systems.

Hydrating upon waking has been shown to flush out toxins, improve digestion, and improve mental performance, as well as greatly improving the complexion of the skin.

The mistake most people make is in thinking that water is the only component of the hydration process, but the fact is, electrolytes and minerals play an equally critical role, so drinking water with a pinch of Himalayan salt, or a salt sole made with Himalayan salt, actually makes sure that your body is more completely hydrated. The electrolytes and minerals make it possible for our body to utilise the water in a more optimal capacity.

A high percentage of water that's consumed in the so-called industrialised west (i.e. tap water) doesn't contain the necessary mineral content to promote optimal water absorption and drinking this mineral-deficient water will, ironically, actually leech minerals from the body, so we end up in an ever-decreasing downward spiral of chronic mineral deficiency. Many of these minerals are difficult to get from the intake of food alone and so Himalayan salt steps up to the plate (once again, pun entirely intended!) to make sure that our body receives all the minerals that it requires.

It has to be said, however, that this isn't necessarily an overnight process, because some minerals that have been lacking over a considerable period of time could take a little while to be slowly replenished in the body.

Chapter 10: Himalayan Salt Lamps

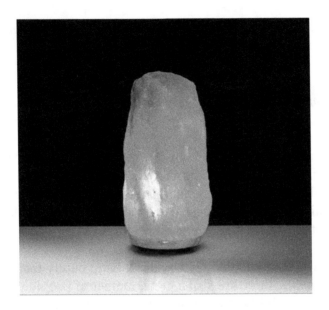

As we enter this section of the book, I think it's important to state that the same stringent studies that have been used to evaluate the effectiveness of Himalayan salt have not necessarily been applied to Himalayan salt lamps.

What follows is largely based on opinion and anecdotes, albeit from tens of thousands of people from around the world.

A few small scientific studies of Himalayan salt lamps have been conducted and some, to a degree, appear to back up the claims of the manufacturers and users, while others seem to give a rather lukewarm reception to their findings. As I mentioned earlier in the book, I very much look forward to the day when a comprehensive, strident, and clinical assessment of the health benefits of Himalayan salt lamps is conducted.

Although the science behind how a salt lamp works is not in question, the reader is encouraged to remember that the degree of effectiveness has yet to be proved - and the degree to which they work is what some scientists still question.

However, there is no debate about one thing... Himalayan salt lamps look fantastic!

Let's continue...

Himalayan salt lamps, also known as "crystal lamps" or "rock salt lamps", are a wonderful addition to any room. The fact that they are a totally natural product and that their colours and varied hues are beautiful to look at are usually enough for most people, even if you put to one side their reputed health benefits.

Although a lot of people may buy a salt lamp purely for its aesthetic value, there are also a great number of people who buy them for their ability to clear pollutants from the air.

This is achieved via a process called "hygroscopy".

Himalayan salt, like most salts, is what is termed a hygroscopic substance. This means that it attracts and absorbs water molecules from the surrounding environment in which it is placed.

Any airborne pollutants, such as pollen, dust, and other allergens that are attached to the water molecules in the air will, by virtue of their actual adhesion to the water molecules, also be drawn towards and onto the salt lamp. The heat from the bulb inside the salt crystal causes the evaporation of the absorbed water back into the atmosphere, leaving the previously airborne pollutants behind, in and on the surface of the salt lamp. This is obviously of benefit to most people, but particularly so to those who suffer with allergies such as hay fever, and other pulmonary function disorders like asthma.

The process as described above has an added bonus in that when the bulb inside the lamp heats the salt, and therefore releases water molecules back into the atmosphere, those water molecules are negatively charged.

The terms negative and positive cause considerable confusion when used in the context of air quality, because things that are positive are usually regarded as "good", while things labelled as negative are thought of as "bad". We are understandably conditioned to think along those lines, but as far as air quality is concerned, you want the environment in which you are living and working to be negatively charged.

Negative ions in the environment have been scientifically proven to reap certain health benefits. Just think of an invigorating stroll along the seafront, a walk in the countryside, being on a hilltop, by the side of a waterfall, or even just taking a shower. All of these activities expose us to superior concentration levels of negative ions.

Have you ever noticed that fabulous scent in the air that follows a heavy rainfall or thunderstorm after you've had a period of dry weather? Well, that scent is the profusion of negative ions that are heavy in the air having been produced by the storm. That smell is so sweet and invigorating!

The actual levels of negative ions can be measured. It's been calculated that air in a countryside setting has up to 4000 negative ions per cubic centimetre, which is about the size of a sugar cube. The air in proximity to a waterfall and the air around a choppy sea shore has approximately 10,000 negative ions per cubic centimetre... but the ion level per cubic centimetre in the air of a busy city can be less than 100.

You can purchase specialist room ionizers that greatly increase the level of negative ions in the surrounding air and the health benefits associated with these have been well documented. They may be a valuable acquisition for many people because exposure to higher than normal levels of *positive* ions has been scientifically proven to deplete the body's energy levels.

The advantage of a Himalayan salt lamp is that its hygroscopic action pulls pollutants from the air, which an ionizer does not. However, it must be said that most ionizers will produce more negative ions in the surrounding atmosphere than a salt lamp. So, possibly the best way forward would be to have both; a salt lamp to help clear the air of pollutants and release a fair degree of negative ions, and a separate ionizer to boost the concentration of negative ions even further.

If you are going to use a salt lamp in your bedroom, as indeed I suggest you do, then it would certainly be wise to leave the salt lamp on during the day to reduce the level of positive ions in the air, as an excess of positive ions in bedrooms has been proved to disrupt sleep patterns. You can then turn it off when you go to bed, as it's also been shown that sleeping in as dark a room as possible prompts and perpetuates the release of the hormone melatonin, which promotes the best quality deepest sleep, during which your body is more able to repair itself.

Although people have been noting for a good many years that having a salt lamp in a room just makes them "feel better", it is only recently that science has been able to show why people feel that way. Once again, it is mainly due to the effect of the greater concentration of negative ions brought about by the Himalayan salt lamp, as this increases both the levels and quality of oxygen supply to the brain. In addition, the negative ions themselves in the bloodstream provide a "serotonin hit", in other words, a boost in the level of the so-called "feel good" hormone, serotonin, which helps alleviate feelings of anxiety, depression, and stress and also boosts our energy levels.

Chapter 10: Himalayan Salt Lamps

It is interesting to note that many people have reported a reduction in the symptoms associated with Seasonal Affective Disorder (SAD) and once again, science is starting to show why people feel this way, as there are a good number of scholars who think that it's due to the fact that the colour of most Himalayan salt lamps, which is anywhere from yellow to deep orange, very closely resembles the natural colours of the sun.

Due to negative ion production, salt lamps are believed to help neutralise EMFs (electromagnetic fields), which are emitted from most electronic devices. This is certainly true of tablets, laptops, and desktop computers, but they are also known to be produced by cell (mobile) phones and TVs, and the health implication associated with EMFs are numerous, including chronic fatigue syndrome, increased stress levels, and a reduction in the body's immune response. Certainly a USB powered salt lamp can be a wise and aesthetically pleasing purchase to help neutralize and counter these unpleasant side effects. I have my slow colour-changing USB powered salt lamp on my desk as I write this book.

As a point of interest, Himalayan salt lamps have been used in tests on children with ADHD (Attention-Deficit/Hyperactivity Disorder) and those with general concentration disorders and it has been shown that the use of salt lamps can dramatically reduce their symptoms after only one week! The symptoms quickly return if the salt lamp is removed. The reason for this is disputed as some specialists say it's down to the negative ion effect, while others think it's down to the relaxing, warm, natural colour of the lamp. I'm quite sure that those who live with the condition and those who are affected by its symptoms aren't that concerned about why it happens, they're just happy that it does.

It is possible, and indeed advisable, to leave the salt lamp on 24/7 because the bulb inside is of low wattage so uses very little power, doesn't get overly hot, and you reap the benefits on a permanent basis.

Replacement bulbs are cheap and easy to source at any local hardware store.

Salt lamps vary greatly in colour due to the variance in mineral content of the area and vein from which they are mined. Some can be quite light in colour, akin to a very faint yellow, while others are of darker shades, ranging in intensity from pink, light orange, peach, magenta, and coral, all the way to deep burnt orange.

The intensity and colour of the light in a room can affect the mood and feel of the area dramatically and is sometimes an underestimated variant. However, its effect certainly isn't underestimated by many businesses, restaurants and hotels, who very often spend tens of thousands on mood lighting in order to get the ambience just right, as they understand just how much the feel of a room is determined by the lighting within it.

We spend so much time in the harsh, white light of an office, or staring at computer screens, that it's a welcome relief to your eyes to have the warm, gentle, soothing glow of a salt lamp in your main living area.

Under the vast majority of environmental conditions, the lamp will not "drip", but in particularly humid environments, a salt lamp may start to "sweat." If this happens, and it really is quite rare, simply place the lamp within a bowl (a natural, low-sided wooden bowl can look very effective) to collect any moisture that may fall from its surface and wipe any residue from around the base with a damp cloth.
Alternatively, you could try placing the lamp on a protective mat, particularly if it's being positioned on a valued piece of furniture.

Due to the action of pulling pollutants from the air onto the surface of the salt lamp, over time it may start to look a little dirty or grubby, which is to be applauded because it's a sign that it's working!

However, the look of the lamp is an important part of its appeal and cleaning it couldn't be easier. Simply rinse a cloth under warm water and wring it out to as dry as possible and, after having let the lamp cool down, gently wipe the surface to remove all residue and restore the lamp to its original colour.

Please <u>do not</u> use soap or any other cleaning product!

Even if the health benefits of a Himalayan salt lamp are of no concern to you, it's worthwhile having one if <u>only</u> for their beauty and the way they greatly enhance the mood and feel of any room in which they are placed.

I don't think anybody ever gets tired of that soothing, warm glow!

Chapter 11: Buyer's Guide to Himalayan Salt Lamps

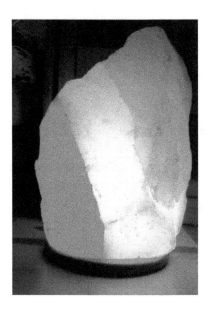

For people who are concerned about and committed to the environment, as we all should be, because let's be honest, this is the _only_ place we get to live, then the purchase of a Himalayan salt lamp certainly falls under the umbrella of "environmentally friendly".

The mines from which the salt is taken are revered by the local people and have been an integral part of their culture and community for centuries. Most Himalayan salt mines do <u>not</u> employ the use of dynamite or blasting of any kind and the salt crystals are mined from the earth manually to eliminate any possible contamination from explosives.

At the present rate of consumption, it is estimated that there is enough Himalayan salt to last for at least another 350 years, as it has been calculated that there are reserves of up to 600,000,000 tons still remaining.

Most salt lamps are manufactured using locally sourced, sustainable wood for the base on which the salt crystal is mounted, but the buyer may wish to get verification of this via the company from whom they are purchasing the lamp. Himalayan salt lamps also use low energy bulbs.

So, all in all, a very environmentally friendly product.

One of the most common questions asked in connection with the purchase of a salt lamp is "What size lamp do I need to buy for my living room/bedroom/dining room etc.?"

It's a fair question when you consider the variance in size and shape of Himalayan salt lamps, which is, once again, down to the fact that it's a natural product, so each one will be slightly different.

Fortunately, the answer is very simple:-

It is estimated that to be fully effective as an air purifier, you need to have approximately 1 pound (0.5kg) of salt crystal for every 15 square feet (1.4 sq mtrs) of floor area.

That being the case, you need to know the floor area of the room for which the lamp is intended, and crucially, that the supplier will send you the appropriate size lamp.

Now that might sound a little obvious, but very often you will find sellers who advertize the weight of the lamp as being within certain parameters. For example, the wording in their product description may read something like, "Weight of lamp: 7-11 kgs" which at first might seem fair enough, but actually equates to a massive difference in relative floor area and therefore, cubic room space that the lamp is having to cope with.

So it's always best to specify the weight you require at the point of ordering, so that the seller can pick out the right lamp accordingly.

Also, it's better to have a lamp that's slightly bigger than you actually need because it will be able to do its job even better if you do… and it's not like you can be _too_ healthy!

If you have a particularly large room and don't fancy the idea of a huge salt lamp, remember that two or, if needed, three separate lamps will do just as good a job as one large lamp.

Sadly, due to the fact that Himalayan salt lamps continue to gain in popularity, partly because of some more recent studies being reported by the media as showing that they have possible health benefits, there has been an increase in the number of fake salt lamps coming onto the market and it's important to know what to look for to make sure that the lamp you purchase is a genuine Himalayan salt lamp that will provide all the inherent health benefits.

Check to see if the light emitted from the lamp is particularly bright, because if it does, it's not always a good sign, as most Himalayan salt lamps emit a soft, warm glowing light. Having said that, it could merely be that the wattage of the bulb inside the lamp is too high, or that it is one of the white Himalayan salt crystal lamps, which brings me to my next point.

Pure white Himalayan salt lamps are quite rare and highly sought-after and, as such, can be quite expensive and carry a fairly hefty price tag. So if you find a white crystal Himalayan salt lamp on sale at very reasonable price, it's more than likely to be a fake.

Himalayan Salt and Himalayan Salt Lamps

A mistake that is sometimes made by the buyer is in contesting the validity of the origin of a lamp that is sold as a Himalayan salt lamp when they notice that the label on the base may read something like, "Country of origin: China". This doesn't always mean that it isn't a genuine Himalayan salt lamp because very often those labels are added at the point of assembly, so it could well be that the crystal is a genuine Himalayan salt crystal mined from the relevant region of Pakistan, but that the base was sourced and the unit assembled in a different country.

Obviously this makes it difficult for the buyer to be certain as to whether or not the lamp is the real deal and in these cases, it's probably best to ask for a certificate of authenticity from the supplier... always assuming that the certificate isn't a fake!

Please also remember that this is a totally natural product and it's not so much a case of "colours may vary", but colours *will* vary. As such, it's usually best to buy a Himalayan salt lamp that you have actually seen in a shop, as opposed to buying over the Internet. I understand that this isn't always possible as they aren't widely available on the high street (yet!) and let's be honest, Internet shopping is so very convenient.

However, there are a good number of reputable suppliers online and if you go down this route, please be sure that they are a highly rated company (preferably long established), advertize the fact that they sell genuine Himalayan salt lamps, that they have a customer friendly returns policy, and preferably that they operate within the fair trade system.

Also, when ordering, please specify in the comments section or as a "Message To Seller", any preferences that you may have, as this could negate any unnecessary to-ing and fro-ing of products between you and the seller.

For example, if you want a very rich, deep orange salt lamp, then please specify this in their Message To Seller section at the point of ordering, as any reputable trader would take this request into account and choose, pack, and ship the type of salt lamp that you requested.

A very simple but often overlooked function of a salt lamp should be the inclusion of a dimmer control. Not all have this option and it's such a straightforward addition to the structure of a salt lamp that I don't actually understand why more of them don't have it. It does narrow down your choice of supplier, but if you're willing to do a bit of digging around on the Internet, you will find a supplier who sells products that offers this function.

Admittedly, you may slightly reduce the health benefits derived from the salt lamp, because in turning down the light, you are also reducing the heat from the bulb, which is, of course, central to the functioning of the lamp from the point of view of any subsequent air purification, but there are many settings in which having the ability to lower the brightness could be really useful. For example, if you're watching TV and you wish to take the lights right down, or in a bedroom or dining room and you'd like to make adjustments from the point of view of mood setting.

In regard to the bulb, it's worth mentioning at this point that when it comes time to replace the bulb, it's very important that you buy a like-for-like bulb, or that you stay within the maximum wattage as recommended by the manufacturer. A bulb with too high wattage can overheat the lamp, and if it's too big, it may come into contact with the inside wall of the crystal's cavity, possibly resulting in condensation running down the outside of the bulb, which could lead to the glass of the bulb cracking.

Chapter 12: Himalayan Salt Blocks

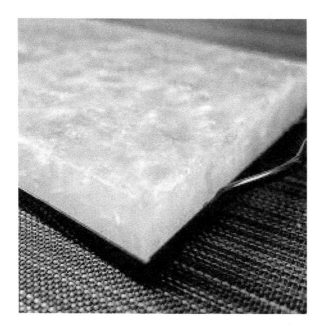

One of the most popular uses of Himalayan salt, due to its inherent stability and heat retention, is that of the salt block for cooking.

As mentioned previously, Himalayan salt was formed under the most intense pressure from the movement of tectonic plates, which means that as a substance, it is quite dense and so has very little space in which to absorb moisture.

This is why it can be carved, cut or sculptured into various shapes and why it can withstand extreme temperatures, hot or cold. It is what's termed a "stable" substance.

A positive outcome of its density, from the point of view of cooking, is how evenly heat radiates throughout the whole block, leading to a uniformity of cooking across the whole surface, and also how the block retains its heat for longer.

Cooking on Himalayan salt blocks, which can also be called "Salt Slabs" or "Cooking Blocks", is becoming more and more popular, not just amongst the "foodie" community, but also with everyday folk like you and I. At this point in the book, you will already understand the many health benefits that can be derived from Himalayan salts, and the use of a salt block is a very sensible, easy, and healthy way of deriving those benefits.

Although most people appreciate the positive impact upon health associated with the minerals and electrolytes found within Himalayan salt, they also, understandably, might feel a little concerned that cooking on a Himalayan salt block will make everything taste... well... salty (!) and that the taste of the salt will overpower the natural flavors of the food. This is definitely not the case because, as discussed, the salt block is extremely dense and, as such, only imparts a hint of salt flavouring into the food that is being cooked.

It is a very subtle enhancement and is in no way overpowering with many people commenting on how much better the food tastes in comparison to sprinkling the salt on the meal just prior to serving. This is largely due to the fact that the subtle flavor of the salt becomes an integral part of the dish during the cooking process, and the difference can be compared to that of cooking meat while in a sauce, as opposed to just pouring the sauce over the meat at the end.

The amount of salt that is absorbed into the food will depend on how hot the block is and on the inherent properties of the food being prepared, in particular, the water and oil content. Talking of oil, if you use oil during the cooking process – I'm a massive fan of organic extra virgin olive oil – then you must very lightly oil the food and not the block, as retained oil could go rancid or even catch fire next time you use the cooking block.

It's important that the salt block is heated slowly, with most manufacturers recommending an increase of no more than 90°C per 15 minutes, even though it's excellent for high temperature cooking as it can be heated to just under 800°C, but a word of caution here:-

Because of its dense nature, and therefore ability to retain heat over a long period of time, it is always best to put the heated block straight onto a carrying rack once cooking is complete.

This can help stop unnecessary accidents because you will automatically carry the block with the handles of the rack, even after it's been left for a period of time, otherwise you may not realize just how hot it still is and pick up the block directly.

NB Please be careful handling the block once it's hot, as the heat from it could easily come through conventional oven gloves.

Bonuses associated with a Himalayan salt cooking block include:-

1. Being a naturally antibacterial and antimicrobial surface, it's easy to clean by simply using a damp sponge/cloth (with NO soap).
2. It can be used as a cold plate for salads and fruit.
3. They are very durable and, with proper care, can last a long time (it's usually a good idea to always use the same side of the block for cooking the food, as this has been shown to make the block last longer).
4. It looks amazing - and even if you don't use it to prepare a particular meal, it can be used as a serving platter.

Only purchase a salt block from a supplier who operates a guaranteed returns policy, because if they don't offer this facility, there's a pretty good chance that it's a fake.

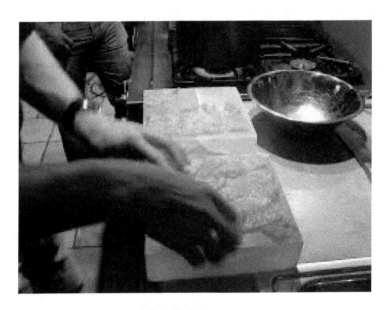

Cooking on a Himalayan salt block

Please always refer to the full manufacturer's instructions with regard to the use and maintenance of the cooking block. This will ensure your safety and help you achieve the best results, and also give the longest life to your salt block.

Chapter 13: Giving Himalayan Salt as Gifts

Some of the gift ideas that you may consider include:

- Tea light holder
- Salt and grater set
- Regular salt lamp
- Cube lamp
- Pyramid lamp
- Color-changing lamp
- Himalayan salt shot glasses
- Pestle and mortar (actually made out of Himalayan salt!) 1
- Fire basket (they look amazing!)
- Night light
- USB salt lamp
- Himalayan salt foot detox dome 2
- Salt lamp globe
- Himalayan salt cooking block
- Salt pipe/inhaler
- Himalayan salt body scrub
- Healing necklace
- Salt fire bowl lamp
- Heart-shaped massage stone
- Himalayan salt massage roller
- Crystal deodorant egg/Salt Ball 3
- Salt bowl for the kitchen 4

1 Use as a normal pestle and mortar to grind a variety of foodstuffs, but the Himalayan salt from which it is made will add a very subtle flavor to the mix. Plus it looks fabulous!

2 The Himalayan salt detox dome works on the same principle as the salt lamps, in that a bulb warms a dome shaped block of Himalayan salt. You then place the hands or feet on the warm, slightly rounded, smooth block of salt, which apparently results in negative ions flowing into your body. Most people report a real sense of rejuvenation.

3 Due to its antibacterial properties, a deodorant egg/ball can be very effective. Simply hold it under warm water and rub between your hands like you would a bar of soap and apply the resulting compound that's on your hands to your underarms.

4 This is such a versatile piece of kit for the kitchen as it can withstand extremes of temperature. Use it chilled to serve up a fresh fruit salad (you'll be amazed at the flavors!) or use it as a baking bowl or casserole dish in the oven... and just like the pestle and mortar, these Himalayan salt kitchen bowls look amazing!

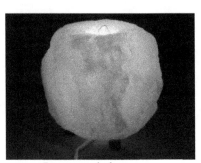

Large salt lamp

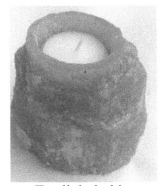

Tea light holder

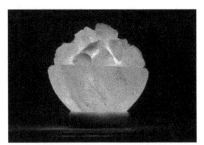

USB powered bowl

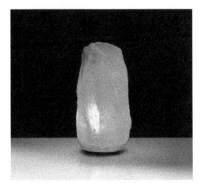

Himalayan salt lamp

Obviously, it's difficult to do full justice to the beauty of all these products within the context of a book, so if you wish to make further enquiries, then please go to:-

www.himalayansaltandhimalayansaltlamps.com

You can click on the appropriate links to any website of interest to you for a more comprehensive presentation of the gifts listed above.

Conclusion

As far as maintaining our health is concerned, there is an almost bewildering amount of advice around, some of which can be backed up by scientific studies, others nothing more than hearsay, gossip, and Internet mumblings.

Some advice, however, is of the highest quality and can indeed be life changing and, in extreme cases, life-saving.

Certain methodologies of maintaining health, both mental and physical, can be extremely time-consuming and expensive. It is the author's belief that it's up to the individual to fully research all aspects of maintaining optimum health, as there are few things more true than the philosophy whereby it is believed that unless you have good physical and mental health, then all others things that you may be striving for, be it wealth, fame, success, material gains, power, or any other relatively transient pursuit, all amount to very little if they cannot be enjoyed within the context of good health.

One of the beauties of using Himalayan salt in the diet is that it's so easy to implement. No big, expensive equipment, no pricey gym membership, no hours of training, but merely a simple and instant change that can reap a myriad of benefits.

I firmly believe in a holistic approach to good health and my philosophy is that the cornerstones, or as I prefer to refer to them, the "pillars" of good health, are good nutrition, weight control, quality supplementation, adequate sleep, moderate aerobic exercise, and meditation. On top of these foundation pillars are a second, yet very important level of activities which include qigong practices/breathing, visualized healing, eye exercises, palming, and acupressure.

Obviously, the consumption of Himalayan salt instead of ordinary table salt would come under the heading of nutrition and it is such a simple, cheap, and instantaneous change to make that reaps so many benefits. It can be done today for just a couple of dollars/pounds!

Not forgetting simply just how great this stuff actually tastes!

The sheer volume of health information can get us to the point where we start to suffer from information overload and "analysis paralysis". When you get to this point, you feel like you're going round in circles, or standing still and getting nowhere and you can even start to lose patience with the whole thing.

However, I firmly believe that every one of us can make significant improvements to our health and future health prospects by making a few simple changes. In fact...

Imagine making a 5% change to your present lifestyle that would lead to a 50% improvement in physical and mental health.

Yes, that really is a possibility and something I've witnessed on many occasions. Making little changes like:-

- opting for organic food when possible
- not drinking tap water, but natural spring water out of glass bottles - not plastic bottles
- cutting down on (not necessarily eliminating) processed food and snacks
- making sure that there's constant fresh air in the room while you sleep, and that the room is cool and dark
- being sure to not be looking at mobile phones, tablets, and computer screens for at least an hour and a half before sleeping
- being in bed before midnight whenever possible

- only eating when you're hungry and eating smaller portions
- switching to unrefined salt
- <u>never</u> consuming anything that contains aspartame (cola drinks, chewing gum etc.)
- walking round barefoot where possible (earthing)
- walking instead of using the car for short journeys, or using the stairs instead of the lift
- getting natural sunlight on your skin for at least 15 minutes a day (don't get sunburn, though)
- <u>not</u> burning petroleum-based candles in the house and not sleeping on memory foam mattresses (the reader is strongly encouraged to research both of these)
- engaging in 10 minutes per day of peaceful meditation
- bringing nature into the home by way of air purifying plants
- occasional yogic breathing

All of the above are very simple, instant, and free or inexpensive changes most of us can make that will really pay off, both immediately and long-term, and are examples of making a 5% change in your existing lifestyle that could bring about a 50% improvement in your overall health prospects.

Now that's a win-win situation and, as anybody connected with business would say, a very high return on investment.

I sincerely hope that you've enjoyed reading this book and that you've learnt something new, or maybe even had already existing opinions reinforced.

Writing this book has been a genuine pleasure... in fact, more a labour of love than anything else.

I wish you health and happiness for the rest of your days and wherever you may go.

Websites of Interest

OK, so you arrive at this page and see just one web address and you might think, "Hmm, not many websites of interest here!", but the reason is very straightforward and is designed to help you, the reader.

The problem is that websites can become outdated, URLs can change, also better and more informative sites can appear or links can become obsolete, but once they're committed to a printed book, there's nothing anyone can do about it.

So the best thing is to simply put a link to my website where I, in turn, list all the links to other sites. That way, if anything alters I can make the appropriate changes to those links and add any new ones as necessary, so that everything is kept up to date and useable for you.

If you're reading this as an eBook or on a Kindle, simply click on the web address below, or if you're reading the printed version, just enter www.himalayan salt and himalayan salt lamps.com, but without the gaps (no need for the http:// bit either!)

http://www.himalayansaltandhimalayansaltlamps.com

All links on the site automatically open a new tab to keep everything simple so that it's quick and easy to navigate to and from whatever you want.

If any new information about Himalayan salt or Himalayan salt lamps comes to light, or the results of new studies are published, I will, of course, add the relevant links to the site for your convenience and to keep you up to date.

Index

Disclaimers

The content contained within this book is for information and entertainment purposes only, and in no way purports to represent professional medical opinion. It should NOT be used as a substitute for expert advice, and you must consult with your designated health professional before acting upon any information contained herein or before undertaking any practice whose methodology is referred to in this book. The author is NOT a registered health professional and the text merely represents personal opinion, not medical fact. The author cannot be held responsible for the consequences of any action derived from the reading of this book, as the content is not based on diagnosis and subsequent regimen. It is the reader's responsibility to seek proper, professional medical advice from a registered health practitioner in connection with any material contained within this book.

Legal Disclaimer (part 1)

Nothing in this book should be construed as an attempt to diagnose, treat or cure. The information in this book is intended to be a community resource. The author takes no responsibility for any informational material or brochures produced using information taken from this book. The author has endeavoured to ensure that all information is correct at the time of publication. This information, however, is subject to change without notice. The author makes no warranty with regard to the accuracy of any information and will not be liable for any errors or omissions. Any liability that arises as a result of this information is hereby excluded to the fullest extent allowed by law.
This information should not be used as a substitute for seeking independent professional advice.

Legal Disclaimer (part 2)

Disclaimer and Terms of Use:

a) i. In publishing this information, the author makes no representations concerning the efficacy, appropriateness or suitability of any products or treatments. Use this information at your own risk. The compiler is not a doctor and has no medical background or training.

ii. Statements and information regarding dietary supplements, books and any products mentioned have not been evaluated by any health authority and are not intended to diagnose, treat, cure or prevent any disease or health condition.

b) In view of the possibility of human error, neither the author nor any other party involved in providing this information, warrant that the information contained therein is in every respect accurate or complete and they are not responsible nor liable for any errors or omissions that may be found or for the results obtained from the use of such information. The entire risk as to use of this information is assumed by the user.

c) You are encouraged to consult other sources and confirm the information.

d) The information you access is provided "as is". No warranty, expressed or implied, is given as to the accuracy, completeness or timeliness of any information herein, or for obtaining legal advice. To the fullest extent permissible pursuant to applicable law, neither the author nor any other parties who have been involved in the creation, preparation, printing, or delivering of this information assume responsibility for the completeness, accuracy, timeliness, errors or omissions of said information and assume no liability for any direct, incidental, consequential, indirect, or punitive damages as well as any circumstance for any complication, injuries, side effects or other medical accidents to person or property arising from or in connection with the use or reliance upon any information contained herein.

e) The author is not responsible for the contents of any linked site or any link contained in a linked site, or any changes or update to such sites. The inclusion of any link does not imply endorsement by the author. The author makes no representations or claims as to the quality, content and accuracy of the information, services, products, messages which may be provided by such resources, and specifically disclaims any warranties, including but not limited to implied or express warranties of merchantability or fitness for any particular usage, application or purpose.

f) The information provided is general in nature and is intended for educational and informational purposes only. It is not intended to replace or substitute the evaluation, judgment, diagnosis, and medical or preventative care of a physician, paediatrician, therapist and/or health care provider.

g) Any medical, nutritional, dietetic, therapeutic or other decisions, dosages, treatments or drug regimes should be made in consultation with a health care practitioner. Do not discontinue treatment or medication without first consulting your physician, clinician or therapist.

h) By reading this information, you signify your assent to these terms and conditions of use. If you do not agree to these terms and conditions of use, do not read/use this information. If any provision of these terms and conditions of use shall be determined to be unlawful, void or for any reason unenforceable, then that provision shall be deemed severable from this agreement and shall not affect the validity and enforceability of any remaining provisions.

i) The information, services, products, messages and other materials, individually and collectively, are provided with the understanding that the author is not engaged in rendering medical advice or recommendations.

j) The information and the terms of use are subject to change without notice. The material provided as is without warranty of any kind and may include inaccuracies and/or typographical errors. The author makes no representations about the suitability of this information for any purpose. The author disclaims all warranties with regard to this information, including all implied warranties, and in no event shall the author be held liable, resulting from, or in any way related to, the use of this information.

k) The unauthorized alteration of the content of this information is expressly prohibited. The author, its agents and representatives shall not be responsible for any claims, actions or damages which may arise on account of the unauthorized alteration of this information.

Printed in the USA
CPSIA information can be obtained
at www.ICGtesting.com
LVHW020039141123
763866LV00036B/739